MW01595180

We are so lucky to have you as our friend and of course doctor. I know it brings a lot of comfort to Ian especially while he is away that we are in such good hands.

Katie Poulter

We trust Dr. Ara with all our medical needs. He is a great guy and a great doctor. Our kids love having him around even when they are sick. Thank you for taking such good care of us.

Emma and Henrik Stenson (European Ryder Cup team member, winner of multiple PGA tour events and 2013 FedEx Cup Champion)

His philosophy on health and wellness resonated with me. I asked for his assistance with getting my entire family on a more proactive path to eating cleaner, sleeping better and living our lives to the fullest potential. The Strickers were good. Now, we are even better. I am so excited that there is now a way for others to reap the benefits of his knowledge and compassion. Thank you Ara, for this gift.

Nicki and Steve Stricker (multiple PGA Tour winner and tour veteran, US Ryder and President's Cup team member).

Quite simply....Ara is the best at what he does!

Ian Poulter (European Ryder Cup team member and winner of multiple PGA tour events)

We are delighted to have Dr. Ara as part of Team Rose. Constant global travelling, trying to be at peak performance and keeping a young family healthy is all made smoother by working with Ara. He is always on the end of the phone to advise on any health issues, and when we are home he checks in on us, saving time, hassle and germs of the trip to the doctor's office. What is essentially a wellness and health service has also turned out to be a huge mental reassurance, and something we value very highly. Thank you Dr. Ara!

Kate and Justin Rose (European Ryder Cup team member, winner of multiple PGA tour events and 2013 US Open Champion)

Dr. Ara's knowledge of the human body is second to none, but how he treats people is what truly separates him from every other doctor. His natural and simple method of treating people with less medication and more holistic remedies makes him the doctor for me and my family.

Hunter Mahan (US Ryder and President's Cup team member and winner of multiple PGA tour events)

There is no one we rely on more for medical advice than Dr. Ara. He has been instrumental in helping me overcome injury, recover from illness and develop a nutritional game plan. No matter what time of the day or where we are in the world, he provides a solution or connections to specialists. He is brilliant. Today I consult with him over every decision I make to help achieve a healthy lifestyle. We are blessed to have him on our team and as friend.

Gabrielle and Gary Woodland (winner of multiple PGA tour events)

Ara Suppiah is the ultimate doctor for 3 reasons: his cutting edge medical acumen, succinctly communicates diagnosis and recommendations at your level, makes you believe you are his only patient in the whole world, and one of the few people I trust unconditionally.

Marty Scirratt, CEO and Founder,
Sync Negotiation International LLC

The first wealth is health and that is what our Malaysian friend has given us time after time...thanks a million!

Ardena and Vijay Singh (World Golf Hall of Fame member, three time major winner and winner of multiple PGA tour events)

LOSE WEIGHT & FEEL GREAT FOREVER

THE INSIDER'S PRESCRIPTION TO TURBOCHARGE YOUR LIFE NOW

By Ara Suppiah, M.D.

Sports Medicine and Emergency Physician

Assistant Professor of Medicine, University of Central Florida

ISBN-13: 978-1482673098
Published by: Ara Suppiah, M.D.
Lose Weight & Feel Great Forever
The Insider's Prescription to Turbocharge Your Life Now
Copyright by Dr. Ara Suppiah, October 2013
Cover Design and layout by Elijah Toten

ACKNOWLEDGEMENTS

Giants whose shoulders I stood on. My gratitude to you is unsurpassed.

- Charlie Ng Say King – thank you for teaching me the art of tennis.

- Dr. John Gosney – thank you for showing that medicine is an art.

- Dr. Steven Saltissi – thank you for choosing to fight my case.

- Dr. Andrew Sama – thank you for saying yes when 352 others said no!

- Dr. Jorge Lopez and my FEP family – for taking a chance on me when you didn't have to.

Giants who placed their trust in me, pushed me to be better and helped make this book a reality. Thank you.

- Vijay, Ardena and Qass Singh

- Ian, Katie, Aimee-Leigh, Luke, Lilly-Mai and Joshua Poulter

- Justin, Kate, Leo and Charlotte Rose

- Steve, Nikki, Bobbi and Izzi Stricker

- Henrik, Emma, Lisa and Karl Stenson

- Gary and Gabrielle Woodland

- Hunter, Kandi and Zoe Mahan

- Marc Wahl

- Marcus Park

- Julie Wunderlich

To my mother Indra,

Thank you for telling me to always shoot for the stars. You remain a shinning example of the patience required for unconditional love, which I test way to often!! I love you dearly.

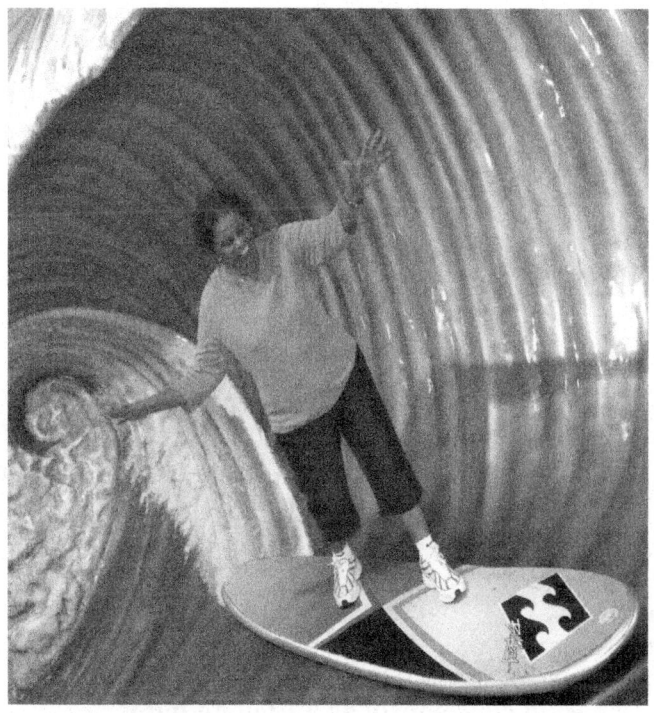

CONTENTS

FOREWORD

My name is Marc Wahl and I am a Senior Physical Therapist on the PGA Tour. I first met Dr. Ara Suppiah in 2004 when we both worked on the Tour.

Back then I was feeling burnt out, exhausted and lackluster. I was frequently sick. My doctor wanted to prescribe medication to control my psoriasis, an immune disease causing discoloration of the skin. I was worried about my health and nervous about taking a new medication.

One day I shared my concerns with Ara. He took an immediate interest in my well-being, developing a plan with me that would change my life. Over the next couple of months, Ara's extraordinary knowledge, skill and commitment helped me transform my body into a well-oiled machine. I went from exhaustion and illness to feeling strong, healthy and energetic. He unleashed what he called the "Viking" in me.

So, how did he do it? No fancy diets, gimmicks or supplements. My transformation was all about simple, easy and painless lifestyle modifications. Because of Ara, today, I am able to meet the demands of my personal and professional life without sickness or medications. I am so grateful to have him in my life.

I have since watched Ara perform the same magic on countless members of the PGA Tour. I can say without reservation that every patient under his care benefits from his skill and learns from his knowledge. His calm, reassuring manner generates immediate and lifelong trust.

Get ready to meet Ara – a frighteningly intelligent, selfless man. This book will change your life if you let it... all the facts and strategies you will ever need for a vibrant life are in here. Even if you only apply 0.01% of what he prescribes, you will be healthier and happier.

Marc Wahl
Senior Physical Therapist, PGA Tour
MS, PT, OCS, Cert MDT

MY QUEST FOR LONG-LASTING HEALTH

When you walk by a store window and see a reflection of yourself... are you secretly a little disappointed that you don't look like a model? Do you try to suck in your stomach or hide behind baggy clothes?

How about your energy level? When's the last time you woke up refreshed and ready to leap out of bed? Do you need several cups of coffee just to get through the day?

Do your neck, shoulders, knees, back or hips ache? Are you on medications for elevated blood pressure, insomnia or diabetes?

Or maybe you have been diligently walking or working out on the elliptical machine but not getting the results you want.

What if – in just TEN short weeks...

You could tighten that belt buckle and start getting compliments on your shrinking figure?

Or fall asleep and stay asleep for eight solid hours, waking up refreshed and ready to attack life?

Imagine being a new you in just six short months – you've become the talk of the town because you literally turned back your clock; inspiring your family, friends and even the neighbors to do the same.

This isn't a pipe dream. It's a promise.

I'm going to show you how in this book, which I have deliberately kept short and concise because I respect your time. You will learn what you need to know and nothing else.

Why? Because this book is all about YOU.

I guarantee this book WILL drastically change your life for the better if you let it.

How do I know this? Because the trigger for my own transformation came from this naked truth: I got tired of feeling like a fraud.

The absence of *disease* does not equal *health*

Why did I feel like a fraud? You see, I am an ER and Sports Medicine doctor. I am expected to understand the keys to good health. I am highly trained with several postgraduate degrees. I've worked in emergency rooms all over the world – in the UK, Europe, Australia and USA. I've also set up emergency medical services in the Middle East and Asia. I've literally treated thousands of people, including numerous world-class professional athletes.

Over and over again, patients would ask me – "What is the key to more energy?" … "Why am I getting sick?" … "Will this happen again?" or "How do I prevent this?" These were legitimate questions and yet I didn't really know the answer and often gave vague explanations that I didn't believe in. I didn't have a prescription that would transform my patients' lives. It's extraordinary to think that as a highly trained physician with numerous postgraduate degrees, I was trained to identify, rectify and prevent disease, but I didn't understand the secrets behind lasting health. And guess what? The absence of disease does not equal health.

I also felt like a fraud because I struggled with my own health. I suffered from periods of weight gain, exhaustion, horrible sleep and frequent colds. Even when I worked out regularly and tried to maintain what I believed was a healthy lifestyle, I did not feel healthy.

The truth is I didn't know why some people were so much healthier than others. That was my question and medical school had not provided me with the answer.

I hated feeling like a fraud. I wanted real answers. I became obsessed with finding the key to long-lasting health, energy and weight loss. That journey took 11 years and took me around the world and back. I kept asking anyone who looked and felt great, "What's your secret?"

Then, in 2003, I had my first breakthrough while visiting my mother in Malaysia. I'd been working out diligently and I thought I was in great shape. My mother, on the other hand, was overweight and had been diagnosed with high blood pressure.

One morning, I offered to help Mom pick some vegetables in the backyard. While my mother harvested the vegetables with ease and grace, I was shocked to find I struggled and quickly got out of breath. I realized that despite her ailments, my 56-year-old mom's body was better able to handle everyday tasks than mine. It was embarrassing: I was busting my gut in the gym and using supplements to build a muscular body, but was unable to carry out basic movements effortlessly. After this revelation, I doubled my efforts to find the key to having both a strong, attractive physique and a healthy body that works efficiently.

I began to study cultural differences and age-old wellness secrets. I attended seminars and read hundreds of books including religious scriptures, which interestingly enough, address the keys to a healthy life.

I applied everything I read about to my body and in the process I became a human petri dish. I tried foods that would make mountain goats sick; herbal remedies that gave me hives; cleanse and detox regimens practiced in ancient rituals by monks, and numerous accepted exercise routines that made no sense to me – purely to see if I could find a formula to lasting health and permanent weight loss.

Life is a grindstone – whether it grinds you down or polishes you up depends entirely on you

– Jacob Braude

It was a long but enlightening process. Eventually, I came up with a formula that provided me with consistent results. Then – in my roles as Chief Wellness Officer for Florida Emergency Physicians, personal physician for many elite golfers and the founder of Golf Medicine at Tour Council.com (www.tour council.com) – I tested it on my patients and my friends. They too got consistent results and were blown away by how much better they looked and felt in just six short months.

Now it's YOUR turn! This book will give you vibrancy, energy and strength that you never imagined. If you let it, my Turbocharge Your Life Now formula will add life to your years and years to your life. I can't wait for you to get started!

Introducing
The Insider's Prescription to Turbocharge Your Life Now

A proven new system that helps you permanently *banish* belly fat, *conquer* Cortisol and *avoid* hospitals.

This book is a distillation of my 20 years of medical experience, research in Western medicine and Eastern philosophy, insight into the psychology of world-class athletes and my personal journey to long-lasting health. The end result is the amazing truth about how to finally feel fit, trim, energized and content for your ENTIRE LIFE.

Before I reveal this exciting system, I need to make sure you understand this:

There's no single "one size fits all" quick-fix pill or routine that can instantly make you slimmer, fitter, sexier, well-rested and more likely to live a long life. Even though we are constantly inundated with promises of quick weight loss, the reality is that despite trying these techniques, we are getting bigger and unhealthier in record numbers. Yes, some quick weight loss gimmicks do work, temporarily. However, most prey on the emotional guilt and desperation of the unhealthy and overweight. We buy into these quick fixes because we are desperate for instant gratification.

However, permanent weight loss requires going back to the basics and giving yourself a realistic timeline to transform your life. That's my goal for you: permanent weight loss and endless energy for life-long health.

Here is a secret that great athletes use when they are goal setting.

Small Changes + Time = **Huge Results**

It took Tiger Woods two to three years to master a swing change. And that's with 10 hours of practice every day. But now he is back stronger and better than ever.

Just like with Tiger's swing example, losing weight, being healthy and avoiding hospitals takes effort and yes, DISCIPLINE. There... I said it. It may not make me popular and I may even risk you not reading another word. I'll take that risk because I have your best interests at heart and I know my method works. Discipline creates habits and the empowering habits produce extraordinary results.

Let's begin this journey with words from the great spiritual teacher Marianne Williamson:

Our deepest fear is not that we are inadequate.
Our deepest fear is that we are powerful beyond measure.
It is our light not our darkness that most frightens us.
Your playing small does not serve the world.
There's nothing enlightened about shrinking so that other
people won't feel insecure around you.
It's not just in some of us; it's in everyone.
And as we let our own light shine,
we unconsciously give other people
permission to do the same.
As we are liberated from our own fear,
Our presence automatically liberates others.

Be powerful beyond measure. Turn the page and get ready for the transformation of your life.

INTRODUCTION:

SAVED BY A SUMO

My life-changing moment is documented in this entry from my personal travel journal. It is my inspiration for this book.

5:51am November 27, 2003

It is a cold bright winter morning in the district of Ryogoku about 20 minutes from central Tokyo. I walk through the wooden doors that guard a Sumo stable. My chaperone reminds me to be very quiet. My heart is pounding with excitement, my palms sweaty in anticipation. I've waited for this rare opportunity for the longest time. There is absolute tranquility in the silence of the stable. It is truly a gift to be here. As I am ushered through the stable, I catch my first glimpse of a Sumo. There he is: a heavy giant of a man with a childlike smile. My heart races and perspiration drenches my forehead. 600 pounds of flesh. He looks strong. And scary. I spontaneously bow and desperately try not to stare! Sumo means "way of the gods" and I can see why.

Sumo wrestlers have been a fascination of mine for many years. I wondered how these small-sized men are turned into giants in such a short time. How and why did the country of Japan, known for its people of diminutive stature, become the epicenter of a sport involving mammoth-sized men weighing up to 1,000 pounds?

The art of Sumo, a 2,000-year-old sport, is fascinating. In addition to size, success in this sport requires enormous concentration, agility, flexibility, discipline, dedication, respect, humility and incredible athletic ability. And a ferocious appetite. Champion wrestlers are hero-worshipped and reach a legendary status in society.

Sumos have a very strict regimen. The junior Sumos wake up at 6 a.m. and start their day by cleaning the stables and preparing food for lunch. The seniors show up about 7:30 a.m. and train until around 10:30 a.m. No breakfast. Their training is extremely physical and highly focused.

At around 11:30 a.m., they sit down for their first meal of the day. It's the same every day: *Chako-nabe,* a lean hot stew made of a variety of meats, poultry, seafood, noodles, seaweed and vegetables. Then comes a boatload of rice or noodles, which is washed down with several liters of beer. An incredible 10,000 calories is consumed at lightning speed. It's a sight to behold.

This meal is then followed by a lengthy nap before the sequence is repeated in the evening.

This Sumo diet has stood the test of time in quickly converting small-statured Japanese men into mini trucks! Unfortunately, most of these guys die in their 50s from heart disease and complications from high blood pressure.

It took me a few days to really comprehend how much the Sumo wrestlers ate. It seemed both embarrassing and fascinating. But what I learned that morning changed the way I approached health and fitness.

Let's take a closer look at the Sumo routine. Why did their daily ritual practically guarantee these guys would gain so much weight so quickly? It's all in this age-old formula:

1. *Skip breakfast.*
2. *Train on an empty stomach.*
3. *Go for 10-12 hours without eating.*
4. *Eat a ton of food.*
5. *Eat as quickly as possible.*
6. *Go to sleep/hibernate.*
7. *Repeat.*

Hang on... the Sumo lifestyle sounded a lot like the lives of many of the doctors I worked with day in and day out... and truth be told, the Sumo lifestyle sounded a lot like my own lifestyle... maybe aspects of the Sumo lifestyle sound like your own life...

It turns out Sumos are masters at manipulating their metabolism. What exactly is metabolism? Let me explain it this way. Your body has a furnace that burns perpetually. That furnace is your metabolism. For simplicity, we will say it is fueled by your body fat. The furnace has a dial that adjusts its temperature. Some actions turn the dial and burn more fat and some actions turn the furnace down and burn very little fat (obesity, starvation, processed foods, advancing age). The Sumos intentionally create a program that slows the furnace down as quickly as possible, causing weight gain. Let's find out how they do it and why it leads to an early grave...

Skipping breakfast.

When you skip breakfast, you lose out on kick-starting your metabolism. You see, digestion requires energy. When you eat breakfast you get your metabolism working. By not eating, you don't burn calories.

Training on an empty stomach.

This used to be a popular weight loss strategy and it does work initially. BUT – over a longer period (three months or more), your body thinks it's starving and it actually slows your metabolic rate. You burn fewer calories, so you stop losing fat and you even lose muscle mass.

Going for 10-12 hours without eating.

Going for long periods without food lowers blood glucose – the main source of energy for the brain. The healthy human body is designed to never let your blood glucose drop below a critical level, so if it's dropping due to lack of food, it mobilizes glycogen (stored glucose) from the liver and muscle to elevate and maintain a minimum blood glucose level. This is what happens during fasting.

Then, when you do finally eat a ton of food, you get a massive surge in the blood glucose. Because there is a limit to how much glucose can be stored in the liver or muscle, any excess glucose is stored as fat without limit. The higher the glucose spike, the more the fat storage. With these cycles of blood sugar drops and surges, you're effectively asking your body to store fat. It virtually guarantees you will gain weight!

Eating as quickly as possible.

Your brain is designed to pick up signals from your stomach as it starts to fill up. From the time you begin eating, it takes about 20 minutes for the brain to send signals letting you know you should stop eating. That's the time it takes to feel full or satisfied. By eating really quickly, you can eat large quantities of food before your brain has the chance to pick up the signal that you're getting full. If you do this on a regular basis you are more likely to be overweight. Nutrition scientists at the University of Rhode Island conducted a study that conclusively proved this. (See the References section.)

Sleeping or lack of activity after a massive meal.

Sleeping after a huge meal does two bad things. It slows down your metabolic rate so you don't burn the calories you just forced down your gullet. And, you store more glucose as fat. You're literally hoarding fat in your body. Talk about being an extreme hoarder!

Before we move forward, I want to be clear that I have enormous respect for the Sumo athletes and this 2,000-year-old discipline. By no means is this book ridiculing their practice. But having a front-row seat to the Sumo wrestlers' lifestyle forced me to realize that many of us, including me, have lifestyle habits that mimic those of our very large friends. Plus, most of us rarely drink enough water… just like the Sumos.

I just explained how dangerous it is to follow the Sumo ritual. In this book I will explain how doing the OPPOSITE will get you back to your ideal body weight and health. In fact, the Sumo Federation in Japan is aggressively pursuing different methods of training to prolong the lifespan of their wrestlers.

CHAPTER 1

THE CORTISOL CONNECTION

When I first started researching the keys to permanent weight loss and long-term health, I felt certain there must be a single unifying positive or negative force affecting us, causing us to gain weight and be unhealthy in record numbers.

For instance, how does the right nutrition make you healthy? Why can eating a lot of processed foods lead to poor health?

How does exercise help? Why is over-training bad? How does meditation help in relieving stress, improving health and prolonging life?

What does adequate sleep have to do with lasting health?

For years I read extensively about these topics, seeking a connection. I interviewed every expert available. I attended numerous courses. But I still could not find the key. Then one day I attended a four-day course by the brilliant high performance expert, Paul Chek. And it was there that I found the unifying link.

The answer: **blood Cortisol**.

What is blood Cortisol?

Allow me to explain it simply. During a 24-hour period, the body secretes both stress hormones (Cortisol) and repair hormones.

These hormones are released in opposite cycles. Stress hormones (Cortisol) are high during your waking hours to keep you revved up. When stress hormones are high, repair hormones are low. Conversely, the repair hormones, released during the evening hours, prepare the body to shut down. When repair hormones are high, the Cortisol level is low.

Here's how it works...

Stress hormones (Cortisol) are released by the adrenal glands in response to light. They allow you to be productive during your waking hours; peaking just after you get up and dropping to the lowest level in the evening. They are also produced in your body in response to physical, mental or emotional stress. It's part of the *flight or fright response*, which is designed to save us from predators by responding appropriately in anticipation of danger.

When it's working normally, Cortisol:

- *Regulates your blood sugar by mobilizing fats and proteins and controlling how carbohydrates are stored in the body*
- *Regulates your blood pressure*
- *Activates your nervous system to keep you alert and awake*

In contrast, repair hormones regenerate our body and help us go to sleep and stay asleep for several hours. They stay low in the blood until around 6 p.m. and then start rising, peaking between 10 p.m. and 2 a.m. They then dwindle down, reaching minimum blood levels just before you wake up. Each day, your body should have a balance between stress and repair hormones.

The following chart shows how this should appear in your body each day. The black line represents a healthy Cortisol rise in the morning and then a decline as the day winds down. The white line represents your repair hormones rising at night to restore your body.

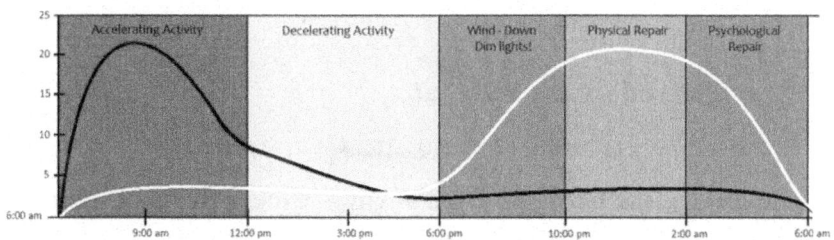

Graph adapted from Paul Chek's Holistic Practitioner Level 1 Course

Now you know how Cortisol *should* be balanced. Here's the next piece of information you need to know: If you have too much Cortisol, it's DAMAGING to your body. The excess Cortisol also reduces the duration and intensity in which repair hormones are released. This means there's less time for recovery from the extra damage. It's a double whammy.

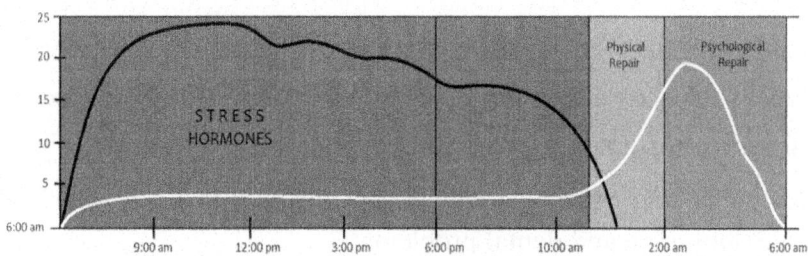

Graph adapted from Paul Chek's Holistic Practitioner Level 1 Course

Let's look at some of the specific, common and scary health problems caused by prolonged and sustained release of excess

Cortisol in your body.

Premature aging and body destruction inside and out

You may look and feel older than your actual age! Your body may experience widespread tissue destruction, muscle loss, bone loss and immune system depression. This includes wrinkly skin!

Overweight and excess belly fat

If you see someone with excess belly fat, it's a telltale sign that he or she has excess Cortisol. Here's why – excess Cortisol increases body fat levels around the waist and throughout the body thanks to a heightened appetite and cravings for sweet, calorie-dense foods and salty, high-carbohydrate snacks. The excess weight is harder to lose because you may also experience huge Cortisol surges at mealtime that increase your hunger and cause you to overeat. As a result, you're likely dealing with higher body fat, lower muscle mass and a reduced metabolism, so you burn fewer calories.

Diabetes

Insulin works to bring down your blood sugar. Excess Cortisol causes your body to become resistant to insulin. When you become resistant to insulin, your blood sugar tends to stay high. High blood sugar can lead to diabetes. Diabetes can cause heart, eye, kidney, nerve, foot, skin and dental problems.

High blood pressure, heart disease and strokes

How many times have you heard that stress is a major cause of strokes and heart attacks? Here's why: Stress causes excess Cortisol which leads to high blood pressure, a major risk factor for heart disease and strokes.

Impaired immune system

Excess Cortisol inhibits our body's ability to fight disease. When that happens we are more prone to both common illnesses like colds as well as more serious ones such as cancer.

Gastrointestinal problems

Excess Cortisol lowers the production of enzymes needed to digest food, which leads to reduced absorption of minerals and nutrients, especially protein. You may be eating the right foods, but because of increased Cortisol, you aren't getting the benefits.

It may also inhibit the growth of beneficial flora (bacteria) in the intestines. These essential bacteria support the immune system, create B vitamins and increase the absorption of minerals such as calcium, iron and magnesium. A decrease in their population results in more colds, sore throats, headaches, diarrhea, upset stomachs and the overgrowth of harmful bacteria and fungus. This will sap your energy, leaving you feeling worn out.

Low energy and insomnia

When your Cortisol is on overload, it means you aren't getting enough sleep and the right kind of sleep at night. Lack of good sleep deprives your body of a chance to properly rejuvenate overnight and consequently Cortisol is not high as it should be when you wake up. And remember, Cortisol gives you energy... when you lack it during the day you experience exhaustion. It's a vicious cycle.

Mood swings and depression

Moodiness, anxiety and depression result from the reduced serotonin and dopamine production in the brain caused in part by excess Cortisol.

Irregular menstruation

Excess Cortisol leads to less estrogen production that can lead to irregular periods. In some cases, irregular periods can make it more difficult for a woman to conceive.

Loss of sex drive

Elevated Cortisol lowers male and female hormones... robbing you of your sexual vitality. You may experience a loss of sex drive and diminished orgasm intensity.

Yikes! That list is terrifying!

And here is even scarier news...

All of these frightening and preventable problems can initially occur without any obvious outward signs or symptoms.

And, you don't need to put the Sumo level of extreme stress on your body to cause a dangerous spike in Cortisol. It happens more often than you think. Check out these subtle Cortisol triggers:

- Working out in the evening
- High volume physical training
- Poor diet (stay tuned… I will explain)
- Food intolerance/sensitivity (lactose or gluten, for example)
- Eating at the wrong times, especially late at night
- Lack of quality sleep
- Environmental toxins
- Trauma, injury and surgery
- Emotional stress, anxiety and worry
- Electromagnetic radiation exposure on long flights or from the use of electronic devices before sleep

You will notice that at the top of this list is working out in the evening. Most of us do not realize the dangers of evening exercise.

Due to longer work days and the availability of after-hours gyms, many of us diligently work out in the evening to ensure we get our exercise for the day. I did this for years after busy shifts in the ER, believing I was doing my body a favor by squeezing exercise into my busy schedule.

But, I was wrong.

When you exercise even with moderate intensity after 6 p.m. (or after you've been awake for more than 12 hours), you spike your Cortisol levels. This leads to an excess Cortisol level at night, just when your body's supposed to be slowing down.

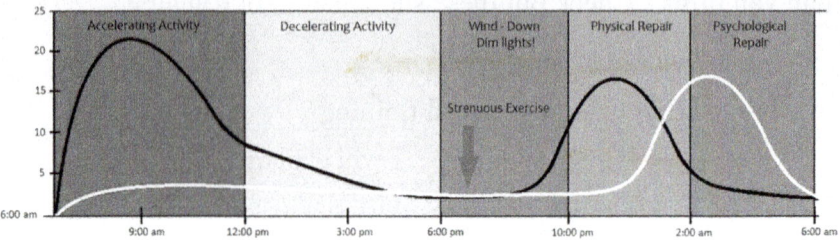

As a result you end up with chronic inflammation and disease… and feeling wiped out all the time. Trust me, I know.

Eating late at night, prior to bedtime, has the exact same effect as exercising late in the evening.

Most people fall into one or more categories of Cortisol-spiking habits and they may not even know it. And clearly, you now understand how the Sumo lifestyle (starvation, overeating, alcohol and long periods of exercise) creates extreme stress on the body every day. It's a major reason why most Sumo wrestlers don't live beyond their 50s.

This chapter may sound like a lot of bad news… but actually it is great news because *Cortisol balance is your key to lasting health*!

This is the secret, my friends. This was my "aha!" moment. Whether it's a young child with frequent ear infections, a pro golfer getting recurring colds and suffering from fatigue, a patient who's not recovering as expected from surgery or anyone struggling to shed excess fat, I now see them through the Cortisol lens, which helps me understand their condition.

The Insider's Prescription:

So that's what this book is all about. Restoring your Cortisol balance! It's a very simple formula you can embrace right now to turbocharge your life. When you follow the formula you will banish belly fat forever. And here's more great news – your body is on your side! You only have to restore your Cortisol balance at least 80% of the time. If you do just that, your body will forgive you for the remaining 20%. If you need to occasionally indulge in a "bad" food or habit, it's OK as long as it's very occasional.

Let's find out how you can get rid of your Sumo habits and take charge of your body forever.

PROGRAM YOUR HEALTH AND WEIGHT LOSS GPS

The road of life twists and turns and no two
directions are ever the same.

Yet our lessons come from the journey, not
the destination.

— Don Williams, Jr.
(American author and novelist)

In this book, I'm showing you the secrets of longevity — how you can stay slim, energetic, healthy and happy well into your 90s.

To achieve this goal I'm going to ask you to take a long, hard look in the mirror to see whether you are currently meeting your own health goals.

Today's *progress* is determined by yesterday's *choices*

You may say, "What? I have a busy life with all kinds of stress and NO free time. How can I possibly find time or energy to get healthy?"

You can, and by the time you finish this guide, you will.

That's because I'm not just giving you a few bullet points about improving your diet or standard tips for sneaking exercise into your day.

No, no... I'm giving you a complete plan of how to easily – and permanently – achieve a healthy Cortisol balance and feel like you can conquer anything!

How to set goals that get you REAL results at last!

We need a clear road to success here... and everyone knows that a map is useless if you don't know your starting point. To get to where you want to go, you must know your starting point.

A wellness self-assessment will help you determine your starting point. The assessment below is provided by the good people at the Wellness Forum. Be honest and answer all the questions to gain a good understanding of your current condition.

And... no matter how you score on the self-assessment, please don't get upset about the results. I'll show you how to start changing your life today!

Part I

Diet

1   I eat breakfast:

Every day	0 points	✓
Most Days	1 point	
Rarely	2 points	
Never	3 points	

2   I eat _____ meals per day

5-6	0 points	
4	1 point	
2-3	2 points	✓
1	3 points	

3   I eat _____ servings of fruit per day

3-4	0 points	
2	1 point	
1	2 points	✓
Usually none	3 points	

4   I eat _____ servings of vegetables per day

8-9	0 points
6-7	1 point
5	2 points
Fewer than 5	3 points ✓

5   I eat _____ servings of whole grains per day

3 or more	0 points
2	1 point
1	2 points
Fewer than 1 per day	3 points ✓

6   I eat _____ servings of legumes per week

5 or more	0 points
3-4	1 point
1-2	2 points
Fewer than 1	3 points ✓

7   I eat foods containing refined sugar, enriched flour and other negative ingredients:

Almost never	0 points
1-2 times per week	1 point
3-4 times per week	2 points ✓
More than 4 times per week	3 points

8   I consume artificial sweeteners:

Never	0 points
Occasionally	1 point
Weekly	2 points
More than one time per week	3 points ✓

9   I consume fast food:

Never	0 points ✓
Occasionally	1 point
Weekly	2 points
More than one time per week	3 points

10   I consume soft drinks:

Never	0 points
Occasionally	1 point
Weekly	2 points
More than one time per week	3 points ✓

11   I consume animal foods (beef, dairy, chicken, eggs, fish, etc.):

Never	0 points
1-3 times per week	2 points
Four or more times per week	4 points
5 or more times per week	5 points ✓

12   (If not a vegetarian) I eat organic animal foods and wild fish:

Always	0 points
Sometimes	3 points ✓
Never	5 points

13   I consume dairy products:

Never	0 points
Weekly	2 points ✓
Daily	3 points
More than once per day	5 points

14   I drink 64 ounces of water:

Daily	0 points
Most Days	1 point
Rarely	2 points
Almost never	3 points ✓

15   I drink the following types of water:

Carbon filtered	0 points
Bottled with minerals	0 points
Bottled w/o naturally occurring minerals	2 points ✓
Tap water	3 points
Reverse osmosis or distilled	3 points

16   I drink alcohol:

1 time per week or less	0 points
2 times per week	1 point ✔
3 times per week	2 points
4 or more times per week	3 points

17   I consume oils (in salad dressings, cooking oils, in packaged foods):

Almost never	0 points
Several times per week	1 point ✔
Once per day	2 points
More than once per day	3 points

18   I drink coffee:

Occasionally	0 points ✔
Weekly	1 point
Daily	2 points
More than one cup per day	3 points

19   Smoking:

I have never smoked	0 points ✔
I quit over 5 years ago	0 points
I quit less than 5 years ago	1 point
I quit less than one year ago	2 points
I currently smoke	5 points

20   Sleep habits:

I regularly go to bed between 10:00 and 11:00PM	0 points ✓
I go to bed after 11:00PM	1 point
I go to bed after 12:00AM	2 points
I need an alarm clock to wake up	3 points
I fall asleep easily when I watch TV or read	4 points

21   Stress:

please check off those issues that are currently causing you stress

__ Children	__ Low self-esteem
__Parents	__Divorce/separation
__Spouse/significant other	✓__Moving
__Work circumstances	__Not looking the way you want
__Co-worker	✓_Lack of exercise
__Lack of sleep	__Financial
__Physical illness	__Not enough hours in the day
__Unfulfilled expectations	__Can't say "no"
__Not time to yourself	

Assign one point for each item you checked above

22   Relationships:

I engage in social activities:	
At least once per week	0 points ✓
Fewer than once per week	1 point

Once per month   2 points
Rarely   3 points

23   Marriage/significant other:

I am happy being single   0 points
I am happily married   0 points ✓
I am happy in a committed   0 points
relationship
I am single and unhappy   2 points
I am married and unhappy   2 points
I am in a relationship and   2 points
unhappy

24   Friends:

I have supportive friends   0 points ✓
My friends could be more   1 point
supportive
My friends are not supportive   2 points
I need to make new friends   3 points

25   General relationship:

Most of my relationships with   0 points ✓
others are good
Some of my relationships need   2 points
improvement
I often have conflicts with   2 points
other people

26 Job/Career

I like my job   0 points   ✓
I like my only parts of my job   1 point
I wish I had a different job   2 points
I wish I had a different career   3 points

27 Personal:

I like myself   0 points
I like some aspects of myself   1 point   ✓
I need to make major   2 points
improvements in myself
I don't like myself   3 points

28 Outlook:

I am very optimistic   0 points   ✓
I am usually optimistic   1 point
I often feel pessimistic   2 points
I tend to be pessimistic   3 points

29 Outlook Part II:

I have a good sense of humor   0 points   ✓
I can sometimes laugh at life   1 point
I have trouble maintaining   2 points
I tend to be pessimistic   3 points

30   Exercise:

Number of days you work out

I work out 5 or more days/week	0 points
I work out 4 days per week	1 point
I work out 3 days per week	2 points
I work out 2 times per week or less	3 points ✓

31   Length of each workout:

My workouts are 45 minutes or longer each	0 points
My workouts are 30-40 minutes	1 point
My workouts are 15-25 minutes	2 points
My workouts are less than 20 minutes	3 points ✓

32   I spend _____ minutes in my target heart zone during each workout:

45 or more	0 points
30-40	1 point
20-30	2 points
Less than 20	3 points ✓

33   I do weight training:

2 or more times per week	0 points
1 time per week	1 point

A couple of times per month   2 points
Rarely   3 points ✓

Part I Sub-Total:_____

Part II

Assign 3 points for every item checked below

Do you often wake up feeling tired?

Do you regularly experience fatigue during the day?

✓ Do you feel that you should be more energetic?

Do you suffer from frequent headaches or migraines?

✓ Are you more than 10 pounds overweight?

✓ Do you have too much body fat?

✓ Does your weight fluctuate often?

Do you experience lack of mental clarity or memory loss?

Do you have problems with digestion?

Do you have gastrointestinal problems?

Do you have constipation on a regular basis?

Do you have asthma?

Do you have allergies?

Do you frequently get colds, sinus congestion or flu-like symptoms?

✓ Do you experience bouts of depression or anxiety?

✓ Do you have arthritis?

Do you suffer from any autoimmune disorders?

Do your joints hurt?

Do you have trouble going to sleep or sleeping through the night?

Are you experiencing menopausal symptoms?

Do you frequently experience food cravings?

✔ Do you frequently eat when you are not hungry?

Do you often feel stressed out?

Do you ever feel bloated or uncomfortable after eating?

Are you taking over-the-counter medications regularly?

✔ Do you take pharmaceutical drugs?

Part II Sub-Total:_____

Total Points:_____

Once you've completed the test and added up your score, let's see how the points compare to the Sumo lifestyle. How did you do?

To get to where you *want to go*, you must know your *starting point*

Under 20 points

Wow! You should have no worries about becoming a Sumo. You're doing a great job! Keep up the excellent work.

21-35 points

Although you're doing many things right, you have an elevated risk of heading toward the Sumo lifestyle. Try to make the improvements you'll find in this guide.

36-50 points

Whoops – you'll need to become diligent and change your diet and lifestyle to reduce your Sumo risk of diseases like cardiovascular disease, cancer and diabetes.

51-65 points

Oh no! You're a Sumo in many ways and your risks are high. Time for serious changes.

66 or higher

Oh, dear. You're a top candidate for the Sumo stable! Seriously, my friend, you're definitely in the highest health risk category, but I can help you. The great news is, you'll benefit the most from my Turbocharge Your Life Now plan. Even small changes will produce huge results.

IMPORTANT! Again, please don't spend even one ounce of negative energy focusing on the results. Remember, your score only serves one purpose – to help understand your starting point so we can get you where you want to go.

Your Health GPS

Next up, let's program your destination on your "Health GPS." You need clear goals to create a strategic and organized plan of action. Why? Because a goal without a plan is merely a wish.

Let's create real, attainable goals based on these factors:

A *goal* without a *plan* is merely a wish

1. Your current level of fitness: Don't plan on running a mile by the end of the week if you haven't exercised at all in a while.

2. Your free time: Do you have one to two hours a day to become

healthy? You probably have more time than you think if you consider utilizing some of your TV and computer time. Plan on giving up a minimum of 30 minutes, five days a week for exercise.

3. Your short- and long-term goals: Pick goals to be measured and reached in six months, but also go for one-year goals, two-year goals and longer. I'll explain why in a minute.

This is not just about weight loss, so take the time now to write down your goals about the following topics:

- Food
- Exercise
- Smoking
- Cutting back on alcohol
- Reducing stress
- Getting enough sleep
- Relaxation
- Relationships

Write down ALL those goals now.

The tragedy in life doesn't lie in not reaching your goal, the tragedy lies in having no goals to reach.

- Benjamin Mays

Do this before you read any further. Seriously, stop reading and start writing.

I want you to write them down because written goals are far more powerful than those you simply retain in your head. I see the act of writing your goals as a contract between your mind and your body. This behavior engages your subconscious to commit to finding ways to succeed even when the going gets tough. All successful professional athletes set clear goals that help them plan their journey to success. You can also bet they don't just carry their thoughts around in their heads. Instead, they write formal plans and review them all the time, just like the destination on your GPS. If you want to succeed, copy these role models.

Here's the secret to setting goals: Be specific about your motivation.

Successful people don't just set goals for the sake of it. They know exactly WHY that particular goal is so important to them. They have such a strong and compelling why that it becomes a daily obsession. It drives their decisions and actions to match their goal. The why of your goal is where the magic lives. For example, one of the secrets of people who remain slim is that they have a number on the scale that they will not go past and they know exactly WHY they picked that number. When the scale reads beyond that number, they take action to immediately correct it.

So, how do you set the whys for your goals?

The "5 Whys" is a system originally used by the Toyota Motor Corporation. It's very simple and really cuts to the core of our reasons for wanting something. The idea is that when you want to accomplish something, you begin by asking one *why.*

Why do I want to accomplish this?

Then, with whatever answer you come up with, you dig deeper, asking *why* to that answer. Repeat this process five times and you will get to the core reason why you want to achieve your goal.

The *why* matters because we often make decisions that are motivated by the obvious reason but not the deepest reason. For example:

I had a 45-year-old patient with this goal: "In six months, I want to be 20 pounds lighter."

When I asked her why, she said, "I want to look good in my skinny jeans."

I then went through the simple exercise of the *5 Whys* with her. Her final answer surprised both of us. She actually wanted to lose weight for a much deeper reason — so that she could be a role model for her family. She wanted her future grandchildren to think she was "cool." The *5 Whys* process helped her establish her true weight loss motivations.

Now let's take a look at another patient of mine and how the *5 Whys* got us to the root of his goal motivation:

Initial statement: "I want to come off my blood pressure medication."

Why Question 1: Why do you want to come off medication?

Answer 1: "Because I hate having to take medication."

Why Question 2: But why do you hate taking medication?

Answer 2: "Because I feel like I let myself down."

Why Question 3: But why do think you let yourself down?

Answer 3: "Because I could have avoided this by being healthier and taking better care of myself."

Why Question 4: But why do you want to take better care of yourself?

Answer 4: "Because when I take better care of myself, I feel good about myself, I'm more confident and feel a sense of achievement."

Why Question 5: But why do you want to be more confident?

Answer 5 – REAL ANSWER: "Because when I'm more confident, I'm able to be a role model, inspire others and make a lot more money."

Wow. That's a lot of insight for a few little questions. For this client, coming off blood pressure medication really meant being more confident and being an inspirational role model who earns more. That's far more compelling than "I hate taking medication." He wants to feel a certain way at the end of the process. And that's what's really important to him. Stopping medication is merely a way to get there.

That's the power of the *5 Whys*.

Okay, now it's your turn to play.

The reason why people give up is because they focus on how far they *have to go* instead of how far they *have come*

Go through the process I just demonstrated and list the *5 Whys* for each of your goals. Actually write them down. When you understand the real motivation, it's going to be easier to stay focused and execute your goals.

Isn't this great?

Now, what else can you do to be even more successful in staying on track?

Easy. Add time frames to your goals in this way:

The reason why people give up is because they focus on how far they have to go instead of how far they have come.

"I want to be skinny at my reunion because I'm going to show off in front of [insert name of high school enemy here] and that means dropping 20 pounds [because, let's face it, I AM overweight].

"I have a year to do that, so I want to be 10 pounds lighter in six months (because I think it will take me that long to get into a good routine) and 20 pounds lighter in a year.

"In two years, I want to remain at that goal weight so I won't have to repeat this process again… ever… as in never again!"

See? Short, midterm and long-range goals… all thanks to clear, specific goals and a timeline.

Now, ask yourself if your goals and your WHYs are reasonable when you consider your current level of health.

For instance, if your six-month goal is to be able to run 15 miles, but you are currently spending your weekends working or dealing with other pressing commitments, you actually have little time to reach that goal. In fact, six months of training for a 15-mile run is a brutal schedule for someone who's not currently exercising or running on a regular basis.

This means you should go back to your self-assessment of your current fitness level and your capabilities… and make sure you put realistic time parameters around the goals.

Remember, no matter where you fall in the scoring results, don't despair. If you've ever seen *The Biggest Loser,* you know that before contestants start the program, they are examined by a doctor and given the bad news about their current state of health. You also know that after lots of hard work, contestants are often able to literally erase diabetes and other health problems!

You can too. I'm not saying that this is going to be easy. Some of the recommendations in this book may feel counterintuitive and move you away from your lifelong practices. The execution may be hard. You may have tried previous weight-loss programs, supplements and diets with temporary success but find yourself back in the same position again. I know that is frustrating. You may even feel like giving up before you start to avoid yet another disappointment. That's when I need you to dig deep and trust the process in this book.

And one more critical reminder...

Please consult your doctor before you start implementing the plans and suggestions in this book. Please make sure you are safe/fit to participate in regular exercise, and follow nutrition advice (including hydration and supplements) in your current state of health (and medication regimen).

At first they will ask you *why* you do it, later they will ask you *how* you did it

CHAPTER 2 SUMMARY:

Set Clear, Specific Goals

- Take the self-assessment to see where you stand now.
- Write down *specific* goals for all the areas of your health and life.
- Make sure your goals are realistic based on your current health.
- Be honest about WHY you want to achieve those goals.
- Make a promise to yourself that you'll make time to make changes!

You can do this! Make this the year you finally reach your goals and say goodbye to your Sumo habits!

Ready to start? Great! Let's go turbocharge your life...

CHAPTER 3

MY SECRET FUELING FORMULA

To eat is a necessity, but to eat intelligently is an art.

- La Rochefoucauld

What roles do food and beverages play in your income, energy and mojo? They play a HUGE role!

What and when you eat and drink can make you more alert, productive and successful OR it can increase your Cortisol (stress hormone) to dangerously high levels and throw your health off balance.

It's your choice!

We all know that foods high in sugar are unhealthy. But what other foods and beverages should you avoid?

Here's a shortlist – I will go into detail about each category in the coming pages:
- Foods that are not ideal for your body type (I will explain this shortly)
- Processed foods
- Food that cause low-grade inflammation from sensitivity/ allergies
- Foods rich in hormones/antibiotics
- Excess alcohol

That's an overview of the basic types of food to avoid, but what types of food *should* you eat to become slimmer and healthier?

What to eat (and not eat) for the rest of your healthy life

I get more questions about what to eat than any other question. It's a topic of heated conversation at many dinner parties. People have very strong beliefs about food, with deeply rooted emotional and cultural connections. And for every person who argues that beef is bad, there are just as many with "proof" of its benefits. Is coffee bad? Is wine good? Coconut milk versus rice milk? What about cow's milk? Vegan or pescetarian? How about tofu?

No wonder we're confused. Every day we're bombarded with information about superfoods, super diets, juicing machines and low-calorie snacks.

We often make our food choices based on convenience, but also based on the latest theories, fad diets and trends – some of which ultimately are not good for our bodies. For instance, the famous "grapefruit juice diet" or the no-carb lifestyles are not good long-term choices, even if they do help with weight loss initially. In fact, studies have shown that an accurate predictor of being overweight is having recently tried a fad diet because they never work for long.

And what typically happens after you try a diet that does not work? You revert back to your original weight or heavier. And why does that happen? It's because of a hormone called Leptin. The more Leptin you have in your body, the more fat you burn. When you go on a restrictive diet, Leptin levels drop and fat burning slows down because your body thinks it's starving and needs to conserve fat to prevent never-ending weight loss. Your body doesn't understand that you are trying to fit into your new pair of skinny jeans so it goes into survival mode. That's why weight loss on fad diets plateaus.

Insider's prescription: Once a week have a "cheat day" and indulge in your favorite foods to keep your Leptin levels high and burn body fat. Cheat your body into thinking food is still readily available!

My research also found that some chronically overweight people develop Leptin resistance. Their Leptin levels are actually high but it can't ignite the fat.

Insider's prescription: Eat natural foods (unprocessed) to turn your Leptins into the fat-burning machines you want them to be.

You see, the trick to permanent weight loss is to reset your weight thermostat through intelligent eating or eating consciously. Not fad diets or synthetic supplements.

But that's harder than it sounds because "bad" food is everywhere. It's simple and cheap. "Good" food, on the other hand, tends to be expensive and requires more effort to find and prepare. Plus, the portion sizes, especially here in the U.S. are far larger than in the rest of the world. Ridiculously huge! So, most people eat what they are served – large portions of non-nutritious foods. And most of us were taught from childhood to finish what's on our plate, whether we are still hungry or not. So is it any surprise that we find ourselves overweight and undernourished later in life?

How is that possible? Easy. We consume calories without any nutritional value. Processed cereals and snacks, for instance, often are packed with calories and chemicals without any significant nutritional value. That's why we can eat 3,000 calories a day or more and still be nutritionally deprived. Our bodies continually crave food to fill that nutritional void, so we have an epidemic of obese people who are malnourished and still hungry.

The simple truth is: Our ancestors, the hunter-gatherers, consumed foods rich in nutrition and low in calories. The foods eaten by most of us today bear little resemblance to the foods our hunter-gatherer ancestors ate. Our bodies were designed to weather the cycles of feast and famine; to accumulate body fat easily in order to survive times when food was scarce.

Thankfully, for most us hunger isn't an issue today. Even when I was completely broke during my first year in medical school and I had to survive on one packet of chips a day, I never came close to the feast/famine cycle our ancestors endured. Most of us are blessed to be able to meet this basic necessity easily and in many cases, in abundance. We have feasts. Feast upon feast upon feast that adds up to a LOT of extra body fat... like the Sumo wrestlers I observed.

Let's stop the madness and eat consciously from now on. This means for every meal and snack, you'll put thought into what you're consuming and what it does to your body, instead of simply eating the food that's readily available.

To eat consciously, you need to follow and eventually master these five fundamental habits.

1. Eat the best foods for your body
2. Eat slowly
3. Eat only until you are no longer hungry.
4. Control your portion sizes
5. Eat three medium size meals and three snacks a day (I know you are wondering what *medium* means — I'll explain this later)

If you wait for the moment where everything, absolutely everything is ready, *we shall never begin.*

- Ivan Turgenev

That's it! If you follow these five habits, you WILL lose weight and enjoy a longer healthier life … I promise.

Take a pledge with me, right now, to eat consciously.

> *I solemnly swear that I will pay full attention to what and how much I am eating during every meal and avoid the distractions that inadvertently make me consume whatever is placed in front of me. Whenever appropriate and possible, I'm going to place one third of my serving in a to-go container for a later time.*

Now let's look in depth at how you are going to fulfill that pledge.

1. Eat the best foods for your body.

Did you know that the best foods for you might not be the best for your spouse? Or sister? Or best friend? It's true. We all have different needs based on our genetics, metabolism, food tolerances and more.

So how do you determine which foods are the best for your particular nutritional needs? These three areas can help: *Metabolic Typing, Glycemic Index* and *Alkalinity.*

Let's start with the first criteria – Metabolic Typing.

Metabolic Typing

To get the most out of your food, you need to eat the food that your body metabolizes most easily.

The right types of food for you *are the ones that YOU can digest easily with very little energy.* That is why a diet plan that one person swears by simply doesn't work for someone else. For example, a lion will not survive on a horse's diet and vice versa. They are both powerful, muscular animals yet they have totally different dietary needs.

People fall into three main types. You're a Carb Type, Protein Type or Mixed Type. Now, does that mean a Protein Type should not eat any carbs and vice versa? No. All it means is that each type represents the foods that give you the most bang for your buck and should make up two thirds of your meals. It does not mean you should only eat that type of food and avoid everything else.

For example, Carb Types digest carbohydrates very easily. Their bodies require very little effort to extract plenty of energy from that diet. They're also the type that feels tired and sluggish after a large steak, because their body spends a lot of energy digesting meat and doesn't get as much energy back. So for a Carb Type, 60-70% of your plate should be carbohydrate. Protein and fat make up the remaining 30-40%.

The opposite is true for Protein Types. They get a ton of energy from a big steak, but doze off promptly after a large bowl of rice. For them, 60-70% of their plate should be protein. Fat and carbohydrate make up the remaining 30-40%.

Mixed Types should eat equal amounts of carbohydrate, protein and fat.

See? One man's food can really be another man's downfall.

Let's figure out your Metabolic Type by filling out the following questionnaire.

The test you are about to take is from Paul Chek's excellent book *How to Eat, Move and Be Healthy*. It is provided below courtesy of http://www.docstoc.com.

Here we go...

Metabolic Typing Questionnaire

For each question, circle the answer that best describes the way you feel, not the way you think you should eat! If none of the answers suit you, simply don't answer that question. If answer A suits you some of the time (in the morning, but not the evening, for example), and answer B suits you other times, circle both.

1. I sleep best:

A. When I eat a snack high in protein and fat one to two hours before going to sleep.
B. When I eat a snack higher in carbohydrates three to four hours before going to sleep.

2. I sleep best if:

A. My dinner is composed of mainly meat with some vegetable or other carbohydrates.
B. My dinner is composed mainly of vegetables or other carbohydrates and a comparatively small serving of meat.

3. I sleep best and wake up feeling rested:

A. If I don't eat sweet desserts like cakes, candy or cookies. If I eat a rich dessert that is not overly sweet, such as high-quality full-fat ice cream, I tend to sleep okay.
B. If I occasionally eat a sweet desert before I go to bed.

4. After vigorous exercise, I feel best when I consume:

A. Foods or drinks with higher protein and/or fat content, such as a high-protein shake.
B. Foods or drinks higher in carbohydrates (sweeter) such as Gatorade.

5. I do best – maintain mental clarity and a sense of well-being for up to four hours after a meal – when I eat:

A. A meat-based meal containing heavier meats such as chicken legs, roast beef and salmon, with a smaller portion of carbohydrate.
B. A carbohydrate-based meal containing vegetables, bread or rice and a small portion of a lighter meat such as chicken breast or whitefish.

6. If I am tired and consume sugar or sweet foods such as donuts, candy or sweetened drinks without significant amounts of fat or protein:

A. I get a rush of energy, but then I am likely to crash and feel sluggish.
B. I feel better and my energy levels are restored until my next meal.

7. Which statement best describes your disposition toward food in general:

A. I love food and live to eat!
B. I am not fussed over food and I eat to live.

8. I often:

A. Add salt to my foods.
B. Find that foods are too salty for my liking.

9. Instinctually, I prefer to eat:

A. Dark meat, such as chicken or turkey legs and thighs over the white breast meat.
B. Light meat such as chicken or turkey breast over the dark leg and thigh meat.

10. Which list of fish most appeals to you?

A. Anchovy, caviar, herring, mussels, sardines, abalone, clams, crab, crayfish, lobster, mackerel, octopus, oyster, salmon, scallops, shrimp, snail, squid, tuna (dark meat)
B. Whitefish, catfish, cod, flounder, haddock, perch, scrod, sole, trout, tuna (white), turbot

11. When eating dairy products, I feel best after eating:

A. Richer, full-fat yogurts and cheeses or desserts.
B. Lighter, low-fat yogurts and cheeses or desserts.

12. With regard to snacking:

A. I tend to do better when I snack between meals.
B. I tend to last between meals without snacking.

13. Which describes the way you instinctually prefer to start your day in order to feel your best and to have the most energy?

A. A large breakfast that includes protein and fat, such as eggs with sausage or bacon.
B. A light breakfast such as cereal, fruit, yogurt, breads and possibly some eggs.

14. Which characteristics best describe you?

A. In general, I digest food well, have an appetite for proteins, feel good when eating fats or fatty foods, and am more muscular or inclined to gain muscle and/or strength easily.
B. I am more lithe of build, prefer light meats and lower fat foods, I'm more inclined toward endurance athletics.

Determining Your Metabolic Type

To score your test, add the number of times you circled A and the number of times you circled B.

- If your number of A answers is three or more than B answers, you are a Protein Type.

- If your number of B answers is three or more than A answers, you are a Carb Type.
- If your number of A and B answers is tied or within two of each other, you are a Mixed Type.

PROTEIN TYPE – Eat this combination in each main meal:

Protein 55%

Carbohydrates 25%

Oils/Fats 20%

CARB TYPE – Eat this combination in each main meal:

Protein 20%

Carbohydrates 70%

Oils/Fats 10%

MIXED TYPE – Eat this combination in each main meal:

Protein 40%

Carbohydrates 50%

Oils/Fats 10%

So now you know your Metabolic Type. Let's tackle the second factor in determining what foods are right for you — the Glycemic Index. I use this to determine the type of carbohydrate to eat for any given Metabolic Type.

Glycemic Index

The Glycemic Index (GI) is the measure of how quickly a food item causes your blood sugar to spike and for how long. It determines how much fat you store. The glycemic index can get very complicated, but I've reduced it to a few basic principles.

- The GI measures blood sugar increase within one to two hours after you eat.
- The index ranks one gram of a food type (on a scale from 0 to 100) based on how quickly it spikes a person's blood sugar.
- As general rule, a 50 or less GI ranking is considered "low," 50-69 is considered "medium" and 70-100 is considered "high."

How does the Glycemic Index work and why is it important?

When a food causes your blood sugar to spike, you release insulin. Insulin lowers your blood sugar by moving the excess sugars into the liver and muscle, or stores them as fat.

Higher GI foods provoke a very large spike in the blood sugar causing a more dramatic insulin surge. Therein lies the problem.

The higher insulin spike leads to a larger and quicker drop in blood sugar, leading to a feeling of lightheadedness, fatigue and hunger shortly after eating. And then, you crave even more sugar. The cycle continues and you gain weight.

Foods with a lower GI rank cause less insulin secretion, less swinging of blood sugar, less hunger and greater satiety, which leads to fewer calories consumed throughout the day.

How can you tell quickly if a food item has a high or low GI? As a general rule, highly processed and sweetened foods tend to have a high glycemic ranking, while less processed foods (whole foods such as fresh broccoli and eggs) tend to be lower in the Glycemic Index. Most non-carbohydrate or low-carbohydrate foods (protein, meat, fat, nuts, oil, etc.) have a low Glycemic Index as well. But there are some exceptions.

For example, watermelon is a wholesome food that has a very high Glycemic Index of 76, but it's high in potassium, vitamin A and lycopene, and low in calories. So it's fine in moderation and when balanced with low glycemic foods.

Here are some other helpful points to consider:

- Glycemic Indexes are based on individual foods, but most people eat several foods in combination within a meal or snack. Eating high glycemic (carbohydrate) foods with fiber, protein and fat will usually reduce the Glycemic Index of a meal as a whole. For example, combining banana (relatively high on Glycemic Index) with peanut butter (fatty and low on Glycemic Index) makes the combination have a lower Glycemic Index. Leaving the fiber-rich skin on a potato will reduce its GI.

- Also, the way foods are prepared (steamed, broiled, fried etc.) will change the final GI number. Baking or steaming will lower the GI compared to boiling or microwaving.

- Be careful! Relying on the Glycemic Index alone may lead to overeating and weight gain. The GI value says nothing about the calorie content of a food item. Peanuts look like the perfect choice with a low GI of eight, but with about 400 calories in a half a cup, they won't help you shed pounds when eaten in excess. So, even with low GI foods, make sure you stick with the portion size so you don't overeat. Portion control is still relevant for managing blood glucose levels and for managing your weight.

So how can you use the Glycemic Index in your permanent weight loss plan? I use it strictly to choose the right foods that form the carbohydrate portion of my meals.

Insider's prescription: Use foods with a low GI to make up your carbohydrate portion of your meal.

I recommend low GI carbs, such as peanuts and apples, especially as snacks and blended in my main meals. And, if you're starving, I recommend a low GI food to avoid a sudden spike in blood glucose, which would cause fatigue later.

For example, these are some of the low-glycemic foods I recommend: quinoa; couscous; brown rice; whole wheat pasta; whole fruits (not juice) such as apples, oranges, peaches, prunes; beans/nuts of any type (but remember portion sizes – these are high in calories), and hummus.

You do *not* want to eat processed, high-glycemic carbs regularly. Generally, this is anything with white flour.

Once you begin to choose nutritious food options without also boosting your blood sugar and storing all kinds of fat, well... get ready for those smaller pants and moving more freely!

Do not let what you *cannot* do interfere with what you *can* do

— *John Wooden*

Here is a list of the GI of common household foods from the American Diabetes Association:

Low GI Foods (55 or less)

- 100% stone-ground whole wheat or pumpernickel bread
- Oatmeal (rolled or steel-cut), oat bran, muesli
- Pasta, converted rice, barley, bulgur
- Sweet potato, corn, yam, lima/butter beans, peas, legumes and lentils
- Most fruits, non-starchy vegetables and carrots

Medium GI (56-69)

- Whole wheat, rye and pita bread
- Quick oats
- Brown, wild or basmati rice, couscous

High GI (70 or more)

- White bread or bagel
- Corn flakes, puffed rice, bran flakes, instant oatmeal
- Short grain white rice, rice pasta, macaroni and cheese from mix
- Russet potato, pumpkin
- Pretzels, rice cakes, popcorn, saltine crackers
- Melons and pineapple

To see a more comprehensive list, the Harvard Medical School website offers Glycemic Index scores for common foods. Please see the reference page in the back of this book for more details.

Alkaline Diet

Now you know your Metabolic Type and you understand how to use the Glycemic Index. Let's move on to the third way to determine the best foods for you — the Alkaline Diet.

The first concept you want to understand is that foods are broken down by the digestive tract to their most basic form referred to as the "ash." The ash of food has an alkaline, an acidic or a neutral effect on the body. I'd like to emphasize that it's the breakdown of food, not the food itself, which has an alkaline or acidic effect. For example, lemon and lime juice are acidic, but their ash is highly alkaline.

Why should you care? You see, the body does not like an overly acidic or alkaline environment. When digested food is either too acidic or alkaline, it is neutralized by mechanisms in the body so the blood stays healthy.

Acidity and Alkalinity are measured by what we call pH level. Our ideal blood pH is slightly alkaline – 7.30 to 7.45 – and the body will do everything it can to keep it in this tight range. Acid-alkaline balance is one of the most tightly controlled systems in the human body and really is a matter of life or death.

Usually the problem is too much acidity and that can cause chronic diseases such as coronary artery disease, acid reflux and gastritis, cancers… and it is a major agent of premature aging, especially of your skin.

So how does our body tightly control the pH?

Acids are neutralized by fat stores in the body – so your body actually creates and holds onto fat to fight the acid. With a constant acidic diet, your body fat and belly fat can't help but stay high to fight the acid. You may lose weight but you hardly shed your body fat.

Whoa – this really woke me up. Not only does excess acid cause most disease in the body, it also keeps your body fat high.

And it's not just about body fat. Another buffer of acids is calcium.

An excessively acidic diet will drain calcium from your bones, causing osteoporosis. Then the calcium will be deposited in the arteries, causing premature or accelerated coronary artery disease.

Here's the bottom line: Too much acid = sickness, excess weight, weak thin bones and early heart attacks.

Now that I have your attention, what should you consume to keep your PH level balanced? Eat alkaline foods daily and generally avoid or reduce acidic foods.

Let's start with the foods and beverages to limit or omit because of their acidity.

- Animal protein including tuna and shellfish
- Dairy
- Processed foods and processed grains especially wheat (even whole wheat)
- Sweets – sugar, soda, corn syrup
- Vinegar
- Coffee
- Alcohol

And what are the healthy alkaline foods? An easy way to remember is alkaline foods are often green and can be eaten raw, including broccoli, kale, cucumber, avocado, spinach, celery and bell pepper. Simple as that. Here is a little secret. Alkaline foods generally tend to have a low GI and are high in fiber. Excellent!! That just made our life a lot easier.

Here's an abridged list of some of my favorite low glycemic alkaline foods:

Vegetables:

Parsley, raw spinach, broccoli, celery, garlic and barley grass

Green beans, lima beans, carrots, beets, lettuce and zucchini

Fruits:

Dried figs and raisins

Dates, black currants, grapes, papaya, kiwi, berries, apples and pears

Nuts and Seeds:

Hazelnuts and almonds

Beverages:

Herb teas, green tea, almond milk, fresh vegetable juice, herbal tea, lemon juice, lemon water, lime juice, vegetable broth, water (pure or mineral)

Whenever I can, I use this list to pick low GI alkaline foods to make up the carbohydrate portion of any given Metabolic Type diet. It's the best of both worlds. I also use it to choose my snacks, beverages and juices.

Metabolic Typing, Glycemic Index and Alkalinity are the cornerstones of WHAT to eat and how to pick your foods. However, we also need to know what foods to avoid, where to look for them and how to become vigilant to so-called healthy foods hiding behind loopholes in food labels.

Let's start with a key principle to permanent weight loss: Don't eat anything you can't pronounce. Stay away from foods that read like a chemistry experiment. That means a lot of salty snacks, candy and "convenience" processed foods are off the menu. To achieve this, you'll need to read food labels and avoid words like sodium benzoate, mycoprotein/quorn or sodium caseinate. Yuck! Once you start reading labels, you'll be amazed at how many foods are filled with chemicals. Especially avoid any product that says it contains high-fructose corn syrup (HFCS) or has trans fats.

The food you eat can either be the safest and most powerful form of *medicine,* or the slowest form of *poison.*

- Ann Wigmore

Here's the skinny on why they're both so bad for you.

Let's start with high-fructose corn syrup which is actually another name for SUGAR. Sugar is the primary factor causing not just obesity, but also many chronic and lethal diseases.

Sugar used to be available to our ancestors only as fruit or honey – and only for a few months of the year. Today, sugar (primarily in the form of high-fructose corn syrup) is added to virtually all processed foods and drinks – even items you normally wouldn't think of as being high in sugar. Tragically, many infant formulas contain more than 50% sugar which helps explain how six-month-old babies can be obese.

Why did this massive shift in the food industry occur? Food and beverage manufacturers began switching their sweeteners from sucrose (table sugar) to corn syrup when they discovered that high-fructose corn syrup (HFCS) could save them a lot of money. HFCS costs about one third the price of sugar. HFCS is also about 20% sweeter than table sugar, so you need less to achieve the same amount of sweetness. It blends well with other foods and helps foods maintain a longer shelf life.

High-fructose corn syrup was first produced in Japan in the late 1960s, then entered the American food supply system in the early 1970s. It can now be found in countless food products including soft drinks, salad dressings, ketchup, jams, sauces, ice cream, cookies and even bread.

Many of us have grown up eating HFCS – and it's the fructose in HFCS that is the culprit. You see, fructose causes massive spikes your blood sugar which in turn stimulates the body to release much higher levels of insulin. Insulin stores the extra sugar as fat and prevents the utilization of these fats for fuel. So the fat just sits there around your belly. Simply put, consuming fructose is essentially consuming FAT. To make matters worse, all this causes Cortisol to rise.

But here's the really dangerous thing about HFCS – the chemically manufactured fructose in HFCS is much worse for you than naturally occurring fructose found in fruits. Studies have linked artificial fructose to about 78 different diseases and health problems, including cancer, diabetes, Alzheimer's disease, arthritis, Parkinson's disease, cataracts and other degenerative ophthalmic diseases.

Yikes. I have another way of describing high-fructose corn syrup: low-calorie poison.

I strongly advise you to limit your fructose consumption.

If you're already overweight, have diabetes, high blood pressure or heart disease (or are at high risk for any of them), you're probably better off cutting that down to a total of 10-15 grams of fructose per day, including fruit, and avoiding HFCS entirely.

Now, the ugly truth about trans fats. Trans fat is made by adding hydrogen to vegetable oil through a process called hydrogenation, hence its other name *partially hydrogenated fats*. Trans fats help foods have a longer shelf life and enhance flavor. They are loaded in many French fries, cookies, potato chips, pastries, pizza dough and shortenings. They are also sometimes in seemingly healthy foods like soups, cereals and granola bars.

So why are trans fats bad for you? Because they pose a very serious health risk, even to children. Trans fats raise LDL "bad" cholesterol and increase the risk of heart disease, and also lower HDL "good" cholesterol. Trans fatty foods tease your taste buds, then they solidify and clog up your arteries.

It's actually better to eat butter than it is to consume the chemically altered fats that are prevalent in junk foods and fast foods. These trans fats are so bad, they're being banned in many countries. The way to detect sneakily used trans fats is to look for shortening, hydrogenated or partially hydrogenated fats on the labels. These are just different names for trans fats.

Insider's prescription: Avoid HFCS and trans fats like the plague.

Loopholes in Food Labels

By this point you are becoming super vigilant about what goes in your body. But labeling laws and some food manufacturers don't make it easy. Reading food packaging labels can be a tricky business, so let's talk about the shockingly long list of packaging loopholes.

Natural

The word "natural" is not regulated by the U.S. Food and Drug Administration. "Natural" makes you think of fresh, wholesome and healthy food, but it actually means nothing about a food's nutritional content, ingredients, safety or health effects. For example, natural potato chips may use *real* potatoes but they are high in empty calories from fat and have very little absorbable nutrients. Natural sugars such as cane sugar or honey still lead to excess body fat when eaten in excess.

Made with Real Fruit or Contains Real Fruit Juice

All you need is one drop (one cc) of fruit juice to justify this statement. The rest can all be chemicals.

Whole Grains or Made with Whole Grains

When you add even a touch (one gram) of whole wheat flour to processed white flour, it can be listed as "whole grain" regardless of how little whole wheat it actually contains. Look for "100% whole wheat," not just the word "wheat."

Multigrain

All this really means is that the product is made up of multiple sources of grain. It does not state whether the grains are refined or whole. Processed multigrains have virtually no health benefits.

Whole grain

You may think a product labeled "whole grain" consists of one type of unprocessed grain. In reality, manufacturers are allowed to use this term even when the product contains a blend of processed grains, as long as whole grain is one of those grains. "100% whole grain" is the only phrase you can trust. Anything short of 100% is misleading.

Fat-Free

Labels that give you a percentage as fat-free can be misleading as well. For example, if you see a label that says "95% fat-free" that still means that 5% of the calories come from fat. Depending on the product, this may be a lot of calories. A better way to assess the fat content is to examine the food label and look for *the number of calories that come from fat and the grams of fat.*

Organic

Organically produced food products must meet standards imposed by the U.S. Department of Agriculture. Organic products must not use fertilizers or have hormones, antibiotics or synthetic chemicals. However, not all "organic" products are created equal. Check out the chart below that explains organic labeling and use it as a guide. It blew my mind!

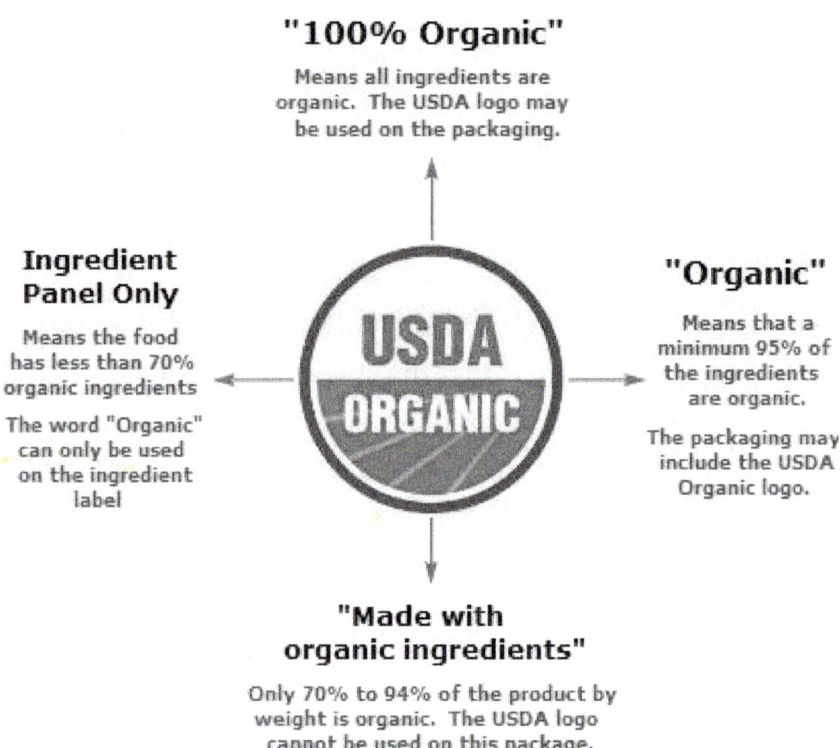

"100% Organic"
Means all ingredients are organic. The USDA logo may be used on the packaging.

Ingredient Panel Only
Means the food has less than 70% organic ingredients

The word "Organic" can only be used on the ingredient label

"Organic"
Means that a minimum 95% of the ingredients are organic.

The packaging may include the USDA Organic logo.

"Made with organic ingredients"
Only 70% to 94% of the product by weight is organic. The USDA logo cannot be used on this package.

Eggs: Cage-Free, Free-Range and Certified Organic

Some cartons say "cage-free" and some say "free-range." Those terms sound great, but they are not as good as you would think because neither has any restrictions on what the chickens can be fed. You want to look for eggs labeled "certified organic." The chickens that produce Certified Organic Eggs live un-caged inside barns and must have outdoor access. They are fed an organic, all-vegetarian diet free of antibiotics and pesticides.

Now you know some of the loopholes in packaging. As a much wiser consumer, you can weed through all the junk to find healthy, satisfying foods.

Okay, now that you know which foods to choose, let's look at the next step to eating consciously.

2. Eat slowly.

At the beginning of the chapter, you took a game-changing pledge to eat consciously. It's not easy, so to help you along I'm giving you five ways to make it happen. So far you've learned WHAT to eat. You determined your Metabolic Type, you understand the Glycemic Index and you learned about the Alkaline Diet. Now we are moving on to HOW to eat.

The number two fundamental of conscious eating is *eating slowly*. If you do just this one thing, you're headed in a powerful new direction. Why? Because when you eat slowly – it helps you eat ONLY what you need and nothing more.

Here are three easy to remember guidelines for eating slowly and getting the greatest results:

- Put down your utensils between bites for about 10 seconds.

- Chew each bite slowly at least seven times.
- Sip water throughout your meal.

Some of you may have heard that drinking water while eating may not be good for you. But here's why I think you should:

- It slows down your eating.
- It stretches your stomach so you feel full faster and consume less food/calories.
- It helps dilute the contents in your stomach and small intestine so that digestion is easier for your body. Think about it like adding liquid to the contents of a food processor — which smooths it out.

Simple, right?

The aim is to get to the 20-minute mark before you lick the platter clean. This gives your brain a chance to process the information it's getting from the stomach.

Eat slowly and you'll notice, perhaps for the first time in decades…

- You feel full way before you finish your meal.
- You actually taste the food.
- You may actually hear or feel your stomach growl as it churns the food.

You *will* consume far less food (calories and fat), so you *will lose weight*!

This habit takes time to establish. You'll have setbacks and that's OK. It takes practice and patience.

Start working on it today. Each time you make your meal last more than 20 minutes, it's a win. Each win will build upon the previous wins to create a lasting habit. Remember the premise of this book: *We're creating permanent and lasting changes.*

Small Changes + Time = **Huge Results**

3. Eat only until you're no longer hungry.

This is the hardest concept in this section. The idea is to eat until you are almost full – which means you are no longer hungry. Not only is this concept very hard to understand, but it is very hard to practice because eating is a socially and emotionally driven behavior. When you're out socially with friends, *almost full* does not come into play. When you're having a bad day and you sit down in front of the TV with a tub of ice cream, *almost full* is the last thing on your mind.

Most of us are fortunate enough to have access to food in abundance so we don't really know what almost full or no longer hungry feels like. If I could modify the human body, I'd ask for a fullness gauge on our belly. But since I don't have that superpower, the following guidelines will help you identify when your tank's almost full:

Think back to the number two fundamental of conscious eating – eat slowly and actively look for your hunger to dissipate. If you are not used to this feeling, it won't be obvious – you need to pay attention. But please trust me, by eating slowly and consciously over time, you will be able to sense the point at which you are no longer hungry. When you feel your hunger subside, you're done. Save the rest for later. You don't need a full/capped tank. This is why you have to master "eating slowly" first.

When you consistently stop eating when you are no longer hungry, you'll notice that you...

- Feel lighter.
- Feel more energetic and awake – you're not using up as much energy to digest and store the excess food.
- Sleep better at night.
- Start to feel hungry within a couple of hours. Cherish that feeling. It's a sign you're heading back to your ideal weight.

The difference between "*try*" and "*triumph*" is just a little "*umph.*"

- Marvin Phillips

Learning how to master this skill won't be easy but it will add years to your life. This was the common theme among the centenarians I interviewed from different parts of the world who were living at their best. They almost never overate. And they ate slowly. Very slowly.

4. Control your portion sizes

Number four works hand-in-hand with numbers two and three.

Do you know an unquestioned secret to a long healthy life? Portion control.

I grew up in Malaysia, went to med school in England and came to work in the U.S. I remember the first time I ate at a mall in Long Island, New York, and discovered bourbon chicken with lo mein and boiled vegetables. A heaping plate costs less than $6. I was on a tight budget, so I was thrilled with this delicious low-cost option. I used to eat there all the time. But after a couple of months, I noticed that I'd get out of breath walking up a hill. Then one day, as I got my fix at the mall, I noticed the weight of my lo mein container and began to investigate my favorite dinner. Turned out each serving was about 1,800 calories! I wasn't eating consciously. I was wolfing down what was put in front of me. Nowadays, I occasionally still order that same dish I ordered in my residency days, but I swap the lo mein for extra veg and split it into three meals.

When you eat an entire bag of tortilla chips, check out how many servings are listed on the label. You'll be amazed. That big bag you just ate all by yourself was supposed to have five servings in it. Oops. Yeah... been there, done that, bought the t-shirt and couldn't fit in it!!!

Here are three proven tricks to eat healthier portion sizes and fewer calories:

Trick #1: Use smaller plates, bowls and utensils. Tests prove that people using larger plates consistently consume more calories than those with smaller plates because there's more room on the plate to fill. In one such test involving ice cream, people given large spoons and bowls ate 14%-31% more than the folks using smaller dishes. Pull out the smaller serving ware in your cabinet and use it! Then watch your calorie intake decrease!

Trick #2: Make a rainbow on your plate. Make sure your plate and food have visual contrast. Interestingly enough, tests show that people subconsciously eat bigger portions when their plate is the same color as their food. Apparently, we are more likely to eat a big pile of white mashed potatoes sitting on a white plate, for instance. Your white dish will work better for you with green vegetables, brown rice and grilled chicken on it.

Trick #3: Remove distractions whenever possible. If you're sitting on the sofa with your dinner watching TV or playing games, it's too easy to wolf down food without eating consciously. In one study, people who actively watched something exciting on television during lunch ate 15% more food than those who sat in silence during their lunch. Savor your food and focus on it! That will make it easier to eat slowly and recognize when you're no longer hungry.

5. Eat three medium meals and three small snacks each day.

You are almost there! We've come to our fifth and final fundamental of eating consciously. This one goes back to a concept you learned in the introduction of the book – when you don't eat for an extended period of time and then eat a huge amount of food, you create a surge in blood glucose. The higher the surge, the more fat you store. That's how the Sumos gained so much weight.

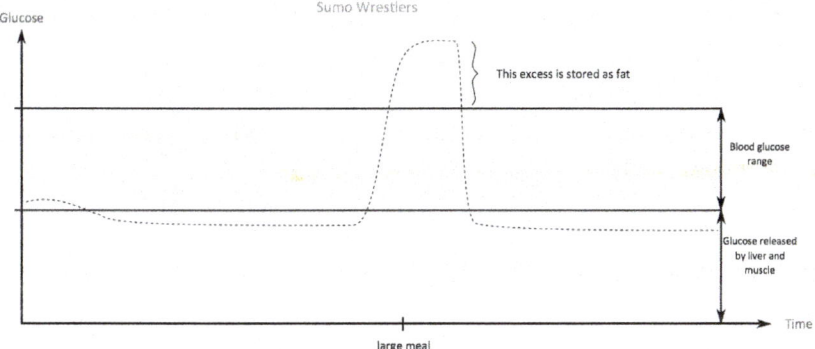

How do you get around that problem? Simple! Just eat three medium meals and three small snacks a day and your body will thank you. You are looking to keep your blood sugar stable and this graph shows a beautiful picture of what that looks like. Cool, huh?

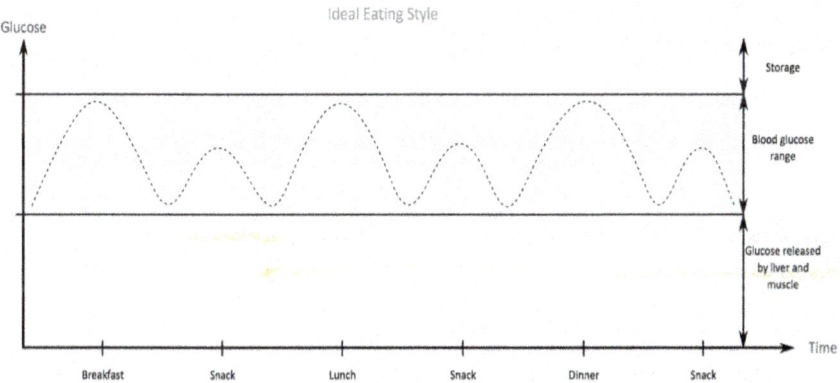

So what do I mean by medium meals and small snacks?

A *small snack* is between 100-200 calories and includes foods like 10 almonds, a banana, an apple, a tablespoon of peanut butter or one egg.

A *medium-size meal* is around 300-600 calories depending on your weight and level of activity. Examples include a peanut butter and jelly sandwich; 16-ounce smoothie with almond milk; a two-egg omelet with vegetables and meat; chicken breast and broccoli, or a small bowl of rice, pasta or noodles with vegetables or meat sauce.

If you're going to eat up to six times a day, you have to eat smaller portions. Otherwise your total calories for the day will skyrocket. Generally, a portion should be roughly the size of the palm of your hand, and no more than half an inch thick. Small snacks are one portion and medium meals are 2-3 portions.

Here's a routine I recommend:

The majority of your energy comes from your main meals, so try to be disciplined about them by following your Metabolic Type. Eat slowly, and stop eating when you are no longer hungry. Pick low GI Alkaline foods for your snacks. That's it! Your energy will explode if you diligently follow this plan.

BREAKFAST:

Remember, you need fuel every morning to kick-start your metabolism. But here is a secret:

Insider's Prescription: Start your day with protein-rich foods even if you are Mixed Type or Carbohydrate Type.

Research shows that people who eat a protein-rich breakfast consume less calories through the day and report feeling a lot more energetic. For instance, have one protein shake and a simple (low GI) carbohydrate, such as nuts and vegetables (spinach, mushroom, tomatoes, cucumbers, etc.). Or it can be as easy as a peanut bar or turkey jerky.

SNACK (Mid-morning):

Metabolic Typing is not as critical for snacks, but Glycemic Index and Alkalinity are. You want Low GI Alkaline foods. For example, choose an apple, a hard-boiled egg or a serving of nuts – you're fine either way.

LUNCH: Follow your Metabolic Type and stick to healthy portions.

SNACK (Mid-afternoon): Same advice as morning snack.

DINNER: Follow your Metabolic Type and stick to healthy portions.

SNACK (Evening): Same as earlier but no later than three hours prior to bedtime!

OK, now you have a baseline understanding of the five fundamentals of eating consciously. These five fundamentals will become your best friends if you let them!

Let's review one more time:

1. Eat the best foods for your body.
2. Eat slowly.
3. Eat only until you're no longer hungry.
4. Control your portion sizes.
5. Eat three medium size meals and three snacks a day.

You can do this – I know you can! And now let's talk a little more about timing because *when* you eat matters almost as much as what you eat. Remember what I said earlier? Eating at the wrong time disturbs your Cortisol balance and saps your energy.

With this in mind, I have two rules – *always* eat immediately after a workout and *never* eat within three hours of bedtime.

I'm not losing weight; I'm *getting rid of it*. I have no intentions of ever finding it again!

Eat immediately after exercising.

The ideal time to eat after a workout is between 30 minutes and two hours – that's when you have a window to replenish glycogen stores and protein to build muscle. This is the best time to eat your carbohydrates especially in the form of fruits, juices or smoothies. Your body is primed to absorb the nutrients and store them in the liver and muscle instead of as fat.

I want you to get this right... so let me tell you about the three common mistakes people make post-workout that diminish the benefits of their exercise.

The first mistake is that they eat too much. You want to limit what you eat to no more than a medium sized meal after a workout. Your body is primed to burn fat after a workout. By giving it just the right amount of fuel, you allow it to continue to burn fat for energy.

The second mistake is to eat fatty foods such as fries or even smoothies rich in dairy or peanut butter. Fat slows down the absorption of sugar and you end up storing the extra sugar as fat. So eat carbohydrates and protein snacks within two hours of a workout and avoid anything fatty in that time.

The third mistake people make is that they don't eat at all. They don't fuel their body when it is primed to metabolize food. Then what happens? Lack of food after a workout leads to muscle loss and slowing the metabolism. What happens next? You hang on to belly fat and can't lose weight!

Avoid eating less than three hours before bedtime.

I know it's tough. We all are juggling many responsibilities and sometimes it's late at night before we finally collapse in front of the TV with a massive dinner. But, please avoid that urge. Eating late at night robs your body of the time and essential energy required to recover and repair. If you can't avoid eating late at night, choose low glycemic and alkaline foods.

My Staple Superfoods, Spices and Supplements

These are my favorite foods to nourish the warrior inside you. Aim to consume them daily.

1. Avocados: Avocados contain vitamin B6, folic acid, vitamin E, glutathione, monounsaturated fat and beta-sitosterol – which all help in maintaining a healthy heart and lowering blood cholesterol levels. They're also a great source of potassium, which helps in controlling blood pressure levels, and are known to help reduce the risk of inflammatory and degenerative disorders. Wow, what's not to love about the avocado? It's truly a super food.

2. Berries (blueberries, blackberries, raspberries and strawberries): Studies have shown that berries can be health boosting wonder foods. For instance, according to one report, women who ate about two servings of strawberries or one serving of blueberries a week experienced less mental decline over time than peers who went without these nutrition powerhouses. Berrics also reduce the risk of Parkinson's and colon cancer. And berries are high in fiber, which is great for your digestive system and regulating blood sugar.

3. Broccoli: Full of fiber, low GI, important nutrients and tasty as well, broccoli is a wonderful food. It's great when you are cutting back on calories because it is full of soluble fiber that helps you feel full quicker and longer and lowers your cholesterol. It's one of the richest sources of Vitamin C, which is a powerful antioxidant, so it keeps you looking younger. It is also a natural anti-inflammatory which protects against coronary artery disease. It helps the liver detoxify the body. Finally, probably as a result of all the benefits combined, it reduces the incidence and recurrence of cancers.

4. Eggs: Despite what you may have heard about links between eggs and high cholesterol, eggs are egg-ceptional for your health. Many people don't know that the 1950s study which gave eggs a bum rap has recently been debunked. Eggs have regained their nutritional value dramatically in the past 10 years. In fact, recent data shows that egg consumers who reported eating four or more eggs per week actually had significantly lower average cholesterol levels than those

who reported eating zero to one eggs per week. In fact, eggs actually increase good (HDL) cholesterol while lowering bad (LDL) cholesterol. Plus eggs are an outstanding source of low-cost, low-fat, high-quality protein.

Now let's debunk another egg myth. For years we've been told to just eat the egg whites. The whites are great, but I am here to tell you not to cheat yourself out of the yolk.

Egg yolk is rich in nutrients that play an important role in overall health and aging. Egg yolks actually contain more vitamins than the whites. They also contain more than 13 important minerals.

Here are some specific yolk benefits:
- Calcium which restores and maintains bone health
- Iron which helps prevent anemia
- Vitamin B complex for brain health
- Powerful antioxidants that reduce inflammation, heart disease and cancer
- Carotenoids that protect eyesight
- Sulfur for healthy hair, skin and nails
- Choline, which makes you feel happy
- Cholesterol to build hormones and maintain nerve function

Eggs are magical – perfect to jump-start your day, on the go or before an important meeting.
Eat whole eggs from a farmers market or certified organic eggs. Up to 10 eggs a week.

5. Greens: Leafy greens are my favorite power foods thanks to

their vitamins, fiber and even their calcium content. They are pure green goodness filled with powerful antioxidants and ideal for a cholesterol-lowering diet. They are also highly alkaline. And they fill you up because they are high in fiber and full of water. For a hearty and satisfying meal, steam your greens with some onions and splash them with olive or sesame oil. Or, eat greens raw… you won't believe how delicious they can be!

My three super spices

1. Cinnamon: This superfood has been shown to regulate blood glucose, reduce the way the body processes sugar (unless you eat excessive amounts of sugar) and prevent type 2 diabetes. Cinnamon may reduce the growth of cancer cells. Plus it has natural anti-infectious and anti-fungal compounds. In some studies, cinnamon has been effective against ulcer-causing bacteria. Finally, cinnamon has anti-inflammatory properties reduce pain from arthritis.

2. Turmeric: This last one may be new to you, though it's been used for over 2,500 years in India to promote a healthy nervous system, control pain and support the absorption of vitamins and minerals. It's a natural antiseptic and antibacterial agent and it's been strongly linked to preventing prostate and breast cancer, melanoma and childhood leukemia. Studies also show that turmeric detoxifies your liver and reduces the risk of Alzheimer's by removing plaque buildup in the brain.

3. Ginger: This spice has a lot going for it. When you eat it,

it fires up the digestive juices to improve the absorption and assimilation of essential nutrients in the body. You can also try floating some ginger essential oil in your bath to help ease aching muscles and joints. Finally, ginger is an aphrodisiac and it freshens your breath!

Dr. Ara's Magic Tea

Want to know how to get a power dose of all the spices I've recommended? I'll share with you what I drink:

Brew some tea (regular or herbal) and add in one slice of ginger (about an inch).

Add in half a teaspoon of cinnamon, a quarter teaspoon of turmeric and a tablespoon of organic honey. My professional athletes enjoy a faster and more complete recovery if they drink this tea when ill or injured.

SUPPLEMENTS:

You'll want to support your well-being and Cortisol balance by making supplements a part of your daily routine. Let's take a look at my recommendations:

1. A multivitamin

Make sure your multivitamin is a whole food supplement *made from concentrated whole foods*, NOT synthetic chemicals. This is where it's critical to read labels and ask your health food specialist. In addition, avoid selenium and magnesium stearate in your multivitamin because they suppress your immune cells that detect and destroy pre-cancerous and cancer cells.

2. Vitamin D3

In a recent study, people with higher vitamin D levels showed the equivalent of five years LESS aging. We are beginning to realize that Vitamin D is essential in numerous vital processes in the body including cancer prevention and immunity. So, the first step is to get your vitamin D levels tested with a simple blood test. The ideal range is between 50 and 70. Most people have significantly lower levels.

Next, where do you get Vitamin D? If possible, it's ideal to get your Vitamin D **from** natural sunlight without getting sunburnt. You can also get Vitamin D in natural food sources such as mushrooms, egg yolks and fatty fish including salmon and mackerel. But for most people, that's not enough – and they will want to take oral Vitamin D3 supplements. The supplements are either cod liver oil or an oil-based D3 supplement. My recommended dose: 5,000 units for adults, 2,500 for children 5-18, 35 units per pound for children under five. Most multi-vitamins do not meet this recommendation so you will probably need an additional Vitamin D3 supplement even if you take a multivitamin. But the key here is to take enough Vitamin D to get yourself in that 50 to 70 range. We all absorb Vitamin D differently, so you need to pay attention to your individual blood level numbers and be guided by your doctor's advice to adjust the dose accordingly. Also, I do want to be clear – I advise a higher dose than most doctors. I do this intentionally because the latest studies show just how important Vitamin D is and I would rather have you err on the side of a slightly higher level because you can't get too much.

3. Ubiquinone/Coenzyme Q10 (CoQ10)

This the fifth most popular supplement in the United States, taken by about 53% of Americans. Why? Because this essential vitamin is beneficial to heart health and muscle function, it recycles other antioxidants such as vitamins C and E, and it's used by every cell in the body. In fact, CoQ10 is also known as "ubiquinone" because it's ubiquitous in the human body. Too little CoQ10 in your body can lead to premature aging, accelerated DNA damage, fatigue, muscle aches, soreness and eventually heart failure. If you are on a cholesterol-lowering statin drug, it is essential that you are supplementing with CoQ10.

OK, we've talked about superfoods and super supplements... and here comes the most basic sustenance of all... and perhaps the most important... WATER!

Let me begin with a story. In all of the ERs where I have worked, I could tell by just looking at the doctors who was well-hydrated. Those who were dehydrated looked sluggish and had the common symptoms of dehydration: Their eyes lacked sparkle and they were often a little irritable. One of my earliest successes as the Chief Wellness Officer for my emergency medicine group was to find ways to encourage our doctors to drink a lot more fluids during their shifts. Their improved hydration made a huge difference in productivity, healthy appearance and the overall morale of our department. That's right, our ER doctors' productivity improved *just by drinking water.*

Water is truly magical. It increases the oxygen in your body's cells so all your systems work more efficiently. It helps clear waste and toxins. It reduces appetite (yes, often food cravings are symptoms of dehydration). Finally, it keeps you looking young by maintaining your skin's elasticity.

So, how much water makes you well-hydrated? For years, we've been taught to drink eight glasses a day, but allow me to give you more current information. Here's my water prescription:

- On days of rest (no exercise):

  Half your body weight in pounds = the ounces of water you need that day.

  For example, if you weigh 150 pounds, you need at least 75 ounces of liquids.

- On the days you exercise:

  3/4 of your body weight in pounds = the ounces of water you need that day.

  For example, a 150-pound person who exercises moderately for 20-30 minutes should drink 112.5 ounces of liquids that day. Most moderate exercisers lose about 1 quart (4 cups) of fluid per hour of exercise, so try to drink about 16-20 ounces of water shortly after your workout to aid the recovery process. To get a more precise number for your body, consider weighing yourself before and after exercise. Ideally, you should not lose any weight but if you do, drink an ounce of water for every ounce of weight lost.

This brings us to the next question, which is, "What exactly should I drink?"

My advice is...

Stick with filtered water and add a squeeze of organic lemon or lime. The magic behind this simple advice is that the water rehydrates your body quickly and helps eliminate toxins. The lemon and lime boost your immune system with a high dose of Vitamin C and neutralize the acids formed from the inevitable stress of traveling, dehydration and electromagnetic radiation. Limes and lemons are my secret weapon for helping patients who have busy travel schedules adapt to a new time zone and avoid illness. I recommend this to all my athletes. And what's the result? They return home with trophies instead of coughs and runny noses.

Now that you know the best type of water, what other beverages are best?

- Enjoy coconut water and fruit juices in small quantities. I say small because they have high sugar content, so keep it under 10 ounces per day.
- Count smoothies toward your daily fluid intake, but beware of what you're drinking! Many of these drinks also contain excessive sugars, simple carbs and coloring. A bottled Frappuccino, for example, has 200 calories and 32 grams of sugar!!
- Avoid sodas and sports drinks. Most of them contain excessive amounts of sugar, simple carbs and chemicals including flavoring and coloring.

- Avoid alcohol. Not only does it make you dehydrated, but it's full of calories, it's acidic and it's high glycemic. Also, studies show that alcohol kills brain cells. If you really can't give up alcohol, stick to just one glass of red wine a day.

And what about coffee? Not one week goes by that I don't get asked about the pros and cons of drinking coffee.

I grew up drinking coffee. I love coffee. I used to be proud of the fact that I could drink coffee at night and sleep soundly. I drink my coffee with a dash of milk, no sugar. So I thought there were really no real downsides to my habit. Then, during my journey of discovery and research into permanent weight loss, I realized coffee is highly acidic. And as we learned earlier, *acidic foods have many negative repercussions.* Hmmm.

At the same time, I noticed both Sardinians and Costa Ricans, recognized as some of the healthiest populations in the world, drank coffee every day. And strong coffee. Way stronger than what I drank. And statistically both populations are healthier than the rest of the world. Hmmm....

Coffee does have enticing upsides. Many people, including myself, enjoy the taste and the smell. It is a stimulant that keeps you alert and makes you feel like you have more energy. It can give you a small jolt when you need it during the day. Coffee has also been shown to protect against Alzheimer's and heart disease.

However, excess coffee can make some people irritable, jittery or even give them heart palpitations. There is also a correlation in some people between coffee and stomach ulcers. That's not good.

Plus, coffee drinkers often end up drinking a whole lot of calories inadvertently. A typical latte contains 200-300 calories compared to 50 calories for a regular coffee with sugar. Even skim milk adds calories. If you are drinking three or four lattes per day, that may be almost 500 calories, depending on the size of the drink. And if you use sugar (either in the form of white or brown table sugar or flavored syrup) you promote weight gain and increase body fat. At 500 calories, a Frappuccino is a dessert, not a coffee.

So here's the real scoop on coffee. It depends on the individual, the time they have their coffee, the amount and what they put in it. People react differently to coffee – but here's one interesting tidbit. Research shows that if your Metabolic Type is Protein, coffee can provide many of the benefits without the downsides.

Insider's prescription: If you enjoy and can tolerate it, up to three cups of coffee a day, with as few additives as possible, is OK. Do not use fake dairy creamers – use skim milk instead. Don't drink coffee in the evening because you will risk upsetting your Cortisol balance.

It's important to note that while there's positive data on coffee and a small amount of caffeine, these benefits don't translate into positive benefits for energy drinks and caffeine pills. There are many antioxidants and bioactive compounds in coffee that are interacting with its caffeine content to provide some value to drinkers. Energy drinks do not have the same potential benefits.

OK, so we've talked about coffee… and we've reached a very exciting point because I've now covered everything you need to know about healthy food and hydration.

Think about what you've just learned. And think about turning it into a fantastic lifelong plan to feel like a million bucks!

This is your new life, starting today – a new path that will set you free from poor nutritional choices... and help you reduce belly fat and your risk of chronic illness.

Your MAGIC FUELING FORMULA

Now you know the formula that's going to kick your inner Sumo's butt!

You learned your Metabolic Type and the importance of choosing low GI foods and low acidic foods.

You have newfound insights about eating consciously (slowly and till you're no longer hungry), plus portion control, food combinations, food labeling and proper hydration.

Now you get to map out your daily fueling schedule.

IMPORTANT! I'm deliberately keeping the specific food and hydration details out of your Magic Formula here, because it truly needs to be customized for your Metabolic Type and all the other factors we've discussed.

You'll pick out exactly what you want – and what's best for you – by following these steps:

- ✓ Get your Metabolic Typing done if you haven't already.
- ✓ Start the day with 500 ml (17 ounces) of filtered water with a full organic lemon or lime squeezed in.
- ✓ Be sure to track your water for the day, so you drink the full amount for your weight.
- ✓ Eat three medium meals and three small snacks each day and include the best foods for your body.
- ✓ Eat slowly, stop eating once you feel full and make sure you control your portion size.
- ✓ Make sure to consume your recommended volume of daily liquids (one-half your body weight in pounds – ounces of liquids required daily). For most people it's easier to drink water gradually throughout the day... but what's really important is that you hit your number.

That's it!

Energy, clarity, a sense of fullness and contentment and good health are all possible when you put these strategies in play. I've armed you with all the food information and a framework for you to create a *winning plan* for weight loss, energy and longevity.

In the next chapter, I'll give you an exercise plan to make sure you're moving every day in ways that are fun and highly beneficial for you!

Finally you will lose weight for good!

CHAPTER 4

JUST MOVE: THE 20-MINUTE EXERCISE SOLUTION

Lack of activity *destroys* the good condition of every human being while movement and methodical physical exercise save it and *preserve* it.

- Plato

What role does exercise play in your Cortisol balance and enjoying life?

- Exercising correctly will reduce and help balance excess Cortisol.
- High-intensity exercise for a short duration is the key to Cortisol balance.
- Avoid frequent long-duration exercise (more than 60 minutes) because it leads to excess Cortisol.

- Ideally, you should exercise when Cortisol is already high – within six hours of waking up.
- Exercising when your Cortisol levels are low (usually 12 hours after waking up, or in the late evening) causes a spike in Cortisol. The uptick reduces the relaxing hormones and impairs recovery and rejuvenation so you don't sleep well and you feel exhausted.

Now let's look at the wonderful benefits of exercising the *right way*.

The human body is designed to move. One of our greatest gifts is to be able to run, jump, skip, crawl, pull and push. After moving, even the most overweight people feel better, both physically and emotionally.

Used correctly, the human musculoskeletal system is a highly efficient machine that requires daily usage (but not overuse). But when you don't exercise you have a serious problem called *atrophy.*

If you're unaware of atrophy, picture this: You have bones and muscles held together by connective tissues. When you sit around at a desk or don't exercise regularly, the muscles actually decrease in size. They pull away from the bone. This process makes your body weaker and frailer over time. Your joints compensate and become mechanically inefficient. They wear out prematurely, stiffen up and ache. Your breathing capacity decreases, heart rate quickens even when you're at rest and you find it tough to move around.

Here's the good news: Atrophy is reversible! It takes more effort and more time the older you get, but it's still reversible.

I know this because I have witnessed first-hand how a well-maintained physical body can perform difficult tasks with great ease and agility at an age when most of us would just be happy to be alive. On the flip side, I'm reminded on every ER shift how obesity leads to atrophy and declining health.

I've seen a 100-year-old Japanese man sprint gracefully. I've seen a 96-year-old Italian lady carry heavy bags up 101 steps on the edge of a cliff. Their secret lies in Newton's Law of Motion, which says that a body in motion will remain in motion until an external force is applied to it.

That external force, in most cases, is our conscious or unconscious decision to quit moving. I know so many people who are riddled with arthritis who would give anything to run again, but physically cannot. I remember seeing tears of sadness and frustration in my grandmother's eyes when she had a stroke and couldn't walk. She, like most of us, took her ability to move for granted until she could no longer walk, instead of cherishing it as an amazing gift.

Folks, tomorrow is uncertain – be grateful for what you have today and make the decision to move. That's it. No fancy plans, no amazing secrets.

You know, one of the great ironies of medical school is that medical students spend years learning how to prescribe drugs, but never learn how to prescribe exercise. Exercise, which has been proven to be the best and most economical medicine of all, is simply not in the medical books.

Check out at all these proven benefits of exercise:

- Reduces the risk of illness and premature death
- Reduces body fat and improves weight control
- Reduces resting blood pressure
- Lowers resting heart rate
- Increases HDL (good) cholesterol
- Decreases total cholesterol
- Improves glucose tolerance and reduces insulin resistance
- Decreases clinical symptoms of anxiety, tension and depression
- Improves heart and lung function
- Increases blood supply to the muscles
- Enhances muscles' ability to use oxygen
- Increases muscle strength

"Wow! That's quite a list, how do I get started?" you say.

Here are the basics…

1. When's the best time to exercise?

For Cortisol balance and optimal health, I advise working out as soon as you wake up. That's first thing in the morning for most of us (shift workers doing night shift may have a different time frame for waking up).

Yes, you have to attend to the kids. Yes, you have a dozen tasks you need to do before you start your day… but my best advice is to take 20 minutes for yourself **first.** It will be hard initially. But do this and you will be a better parent, spouse and employee. You set up your day to WIN. And you'll lead by example.... you owe that to yourself and your family!!

Why exercise first thing in the morning? No, there's no magical energy force between the hours of 6 a.m. and 9 a.m. that pulls fat from the body or "rips the abs." It's simply that the hours after you wake up provide a few golden opportunities that are not as powerful later in the day. Take a look...

- If you get your metabolism cranked up in the morning by exercising, it can often remain at an elevated level throughout the day (even for 24 hours). This means more calories get burned, for free!
- When you wake up, your Cortisol levels are starting to rise. Exercising at that time helps boost your Cortisol without increasing your overall Cortisol level for the day.
- You'll avoid the "Cortisol rush" that night workouts create. As you learned earlier, evening exercise leads to elevated Cortisol, which is inflammatory and will interfere in your body's natural rhythms of recovery and repair.
- High-intensity exercise for short periods of time gives you a mental boost that may last for up to 10 hours. So, work out when you get up and you can be a super genius all day!
- It makes you eat less, naturally. Yes, it's true that those who exercise in the morning find they have far fewer cravings during the day and eat less.
- You're more likely to commit and stick with your exercise routine. More than 90% of people who do morning workouts stick with their program. This is because very few things interfere with it and you can really use that free time to your

advantage!

- It leads to better sleep. Exercising regularly each day leads to improved sleep at night, which means it will get easier to get up to do morning fitness routines.

IMPORTANT! Don't exercise on an empty stomach! Remember my Sumo friends? In the morning, your body has gone eight-plus hours since eating or drinking anything. Your blood sugar levels are lower and your body doesn't have adequate fuel to work out optimally.

Exercise first thing in the morning, before your brain figures out what you're doing

I know there are strong advocates of working out first thing in the morning on an empty stomach. These advocates believe you will utilize fat stored overnight as an energy source since you are not putting new food into your body. In reality, it is nearly impossible to work out with significant intensity having fasted overnight. You also risk getting sick and injured. Plus, eating breakfast in the morning boosts your metabolism, but exercising on an empty stomach slows it down. When you exercise without eating, your body does not burn fat efficiently.

For most people I suggest eating approximately 100-200 calories (for example, two hard-boiled eggs or a protein shake or 100% wheat toast with peanut butter) 30-45 minutes prior to exercising.

If you simply cannot work out at all when you wake up, please try to make time during the first six hours you are awake. However, if you make it till evening and you are tempted to work out, remember what I taught you – I strongly discourage exercising after sundown or after you have been awake for 12 hours. Why? Remember what we talked about in chapter one? Evening is when your Cortisol should be declining. If you work out, it increases your Cortisol, leading to less time for your body to recover and recuperate from your day. Give yourself a break and recommit to working out earlier the next day.

Insider's Prescription: Exercise first thing in the morning and avoid exercise after sundown.

2. How long should I work out each day?

Now that you know when you should work out, let's talk about how much. For most of us, **not having enough time** is our biggest excuse. Those who believe they need to exercise for more than 20 minutes every day usually abandon their routine fairly quickly.

Behold! I bring you great news!

The myth that more exercise is better for overall health and longevity… is false.

You're far better off *exercising at a high intensity for a much shorter duration*.

Now doesn't that put a smile on your face?

I work out at least five days a week. People think it's because I love it. I don't! I drag myself to the gym like everyone else. It's a necessary evil, but I always feel good afterwards. It keeps me mentally sharp and my energy levels high. A full hour, though, was tough to spare.

So you can imagine how ecstatic I was when I found I could get the maximum benefits of exercise in just 20 minutes a day! Now, that's all I do most days!

There's a ton of evidence to support short high-intensity interval training, but here are just a few key findings to consider:

- Evidence shows that high-intensity interval training requires a mere fraction of the time AND is FAR more efficient and effective. When it comes to exercise, more is not always better. The same can be said for the super-slow form of weight training.
- Interval training can dramatically improve your cardiovascular fitness and fat-burning capabilities in a fraction of the time.
- High-intensity exercise not only boosts fat burning but also automatically helps create muscle definition all over your body.
- Recent evidence indicates that long-distance running is one of the hardest types of exercise for your body – and one of the least efficient. A couple of studies even found that long-distance running puts undue stress on the heart.
- The best fitness regimen mimics the movements of our hunter-gatherer ancestors. It includes short bursts of high-intensity activities, but not long-distance running. This is

also how young children and animals move – in short but intense spurts with rest in between.

In addition to all this scientific evidence, here's a candid observation from working in the hospitals and with athletes: I generally don't see an overweight long distance runner – however, they sometimes look as if the years of stress on their body have taken its toll. *Your body's optimal workout is short bursts of high-intensity exercise with rest and recuperation in between.* It's something to consider!

With all this evidence, here's what I advocate:

If you're looking for the minimum required dose of exercise to keep you healthy, keep your heart strong and help you sleep at night – shorter and more intense is the way to go.

If you haven't been exercising regularly, I recommend you exercise 20 minutes per day, five days a week, as soon as you wake up.

If you already regularly exercise, consider my routine below as a way to get the most benefit with the minimum time required.

3. What are the best exercises to do?

Now that you know when and how much, let's talk about HOW you should actually exercise.

Remember, our aim is to improve your health and well-being.

To do that, you need to follow a varied and balanced fitness program that incorporates four types of exercise/movements suitable to your current level of fitness. Plus, you have to shake it up regularly. Variety keeps your body and mind adaptable and flexible. Variety also stimulates muscle growth, engages the mind and slows premature aging.

These are the four types of exercises:

1. High-Intensity Interval Training (HIIT) for maximum cardiovascular benefits.

2. Strength/Resistance Training to stimulate muscle growth and maintain joint function.

3. Core Exercises to support activities of daily living, maintain great posture and prevent lower back pain.

4. Stretching to keep joints supple, muscles strong, and tendons and ligaments pliable to prevent injuries.

Let's look at each type.

1. High-Intensity Interval Training (HIIT)

I want you to get the biggest bang for your buck. Therefore, even for a novice, high-intensity interval training is the most effective and efficient form of exercise because it works your aerobic (using oxygen) AND anaerobic (without oxygen) processes for optimal cardiovascular benefit.

No matter how slow you go, you are still lapping everyone on the couch

HIIT may sound like a scary prospect especially if your idea of exercise is walking from the couch to the fridge and back. I get that. But the core principle of HIIT is actually very simple: Move as quickly as you can in short bursts. When intensity is high, you don't work out more than 20 minutes, but you still get all the benefits of a longer workout.

So to build a high-intensity workout, keep the FITT principles in mind (Frequency, Intensity, Type and Time).

Frequency

You want to do HITT a maximum of three days per week with at least one day off between sessions.

IMPORTANT REST MANDATE!

If you're following a HIIT routine, you must obey two rules:

First, *do not* do this more than three times a week,

Second, *do not* do this on consecutive days. Have a rest on the days in-between.

Doing a HIIT routine more frequently risks injury, spiking your

Cortisol, wearing down your body and making it more susceptible to illness. Never ever do HIIT back-to-back on consecutive days.

There are plenty of *obstacles* in your path.
Don't allow yourself to become one of them.

- Ralph Marston

Intensity

It's common to struggle with finding the right intensity, so let me help you figure that out. Picture this: You are walking up a hill at a slow leisurely pace with your dog and you get to the top. You are still able to hold a conversation and are barely out of breath. You just walked up that hill at *very low intensity*. Leisurely walking is a form of very low intensity exercise. Most of us can walk for an hour at a pace that never leaves us out of breath even though we may be fatigued. If you walked up the hill faster and at the end you were still able to talk, but were out of breath between sentences, you just doubled or tripled your intensity.

Now picture this: If you sprinted as fast as possible, most of you would not be able to run for more than 30-60 seconds. You would stop because you'd be short of breath, gasping for air. That is *high intensity*. When it comes to exercise, the best way to reap maximum benefits in the shortest time is by doing high-intensity interval training. That means doing an exercise or movement as quickly and as hard as possible for 30 seconds to one minute that leaves you gasping for air. Then take the time to fully recover before doing the exercise again at the same intensity. You repeat this process (interval) as many times as possible in a 20-minute window. Now, for those of you who don't exercise regularly, it may be that walking at a brisk pace leaves you gasping for air. If this is the case, a brisk walk is the perfect exercise for you.

Let me clarify: Walking is wonderful. In fact, one of my fondest childhood memories is going on evening walks with my family while my grandmother would share stories. It has been shown to make you live longer by reducing stress. If you are not physically active at all, it is a great place to start. Walking is absolutely better than doing nothing. However, for the purpose of long-term health and aging gracefully, you want to work your way up to exercises that are far more intense than walking.

Remember what I said at the beginning of the book:

Small Changes + Time = **Huge Results**

Type

Well, here's another place where that really applies. Start looking for ways to add intensity to everyday aspects of your life. For example, if you're using the stairs, go up and down as fast as you can for 30 seconds. If you are cleaning, pick up the pace. Does it take you 20 minutes to vacuum? Do it in 12! Do you rake the yard in an hour? Do it in half the time! You define what high intensity is for you at any given task and your heart will thank you.

Here are some other ideas for simple exercise you can do at home:

- Walking (if you are returning to an exercise routine or have never exercised formally before)
- Running up and down the stairs
- Running/sprinting up and down your driveway
- Jumping rope
- Push-ups
- Chin-ups
- Jumping jacks
- Twenty Tens (see below)

If you work out in the gym, you can add sprints on a stationary bikes, treadmills, steppers and elliptical machines to your routine.

Fitness happens at every size

I am very aware that finding time for exercise is our biggest challenge. So I highly encourage you to find ways to squeeze in a workout whenever you can. If all else fails, there is a four-minute routine that you can do pretty much anywhere at any time, called *Twenty Tens*. At least give yourself the gift of this short routine in the morning. It will kick-start your metabolism, pump your blood around your whole body and really wake you up so you can be your best for the rest of the day.

If you only do one exercise, this would be it – it takes four minutes and requires no equipment. And it pushes you mentally so you start the day with a win. I do this at least once a day. Starting in a standing position with feet shoulder-width apart, and get down to a squatting position while swinging your arm forward. Then get straight back up to the standing position. Do this for 20 squats. On the twentieth squat hold the squat position for 10 seconds. Repeat the sequence again five times with one modification: Widen the space between your feet by three to four inches each time. This makes it harder. Swinging your arm faster makes it easier. A professional demonstration of the Twenty Tens exercise is available on my website www.DrAraOnCall.com

It doesn't *get easier,* you just *get stronger*

Warning: This is hard. I could not do the full five sets when I first started. Start slowly based on *whatever high intensity is for you.* You may only be able to do three squats and catch your breath when you first start. Maybe you can only do two sets. That's okay. Just start. Build up slowly. Remember, the race is long, and the end, it's only with yourself. So run your own race. .

And remember, Twenty Tens are not a replacement for my exercise formula. I am simply suggesting them as a quick solution when four minutes is all you can spare.

Time

This one is simple, no more than 20 minutes. Trust me, if you are pushing it as hard as you can for 30 seconds to a minute, you will be beat after 20 minutes.

Here's an example of a 20-minute routine – remember to modify it based on your fitness level.

- Warm up for three minutes: At half your maximum speed, do jumping jacks, run on the spot, walk up stairs, jump rope, do lunges or ride your bike.
- Exercise (sprint/run/walk/pedal) as hard and fast as you can for 30 seconds. If you feel it's too easy, crank up the resistance on your bike, elliptical or stair climber to a challenging level or increase the incline on your treadmill. You'll burn twice the calories at a 5% incline in the same amount of time.
- Recover for 90 seconds, still moving (do not stop moving), but at a slower pace and decreased resistance.
- Repeat steps 2 and 3 (high-intensity exercise and recovery) for a total of seven repetitions.

You're done! Cross exercise off your to-do list!
How awesome is that?

Someone who is busier than you is working out *right now*

WARNING! Over-exercising could do more harm than good. It's *not* recommended to do high-intensity exercises more than three times a week. Don't get overexcited as you see results and think you should do this every day. If you do that, you'll totally throw your Cortisol off balance by overtraining and miss out on the benefits. That's why I repeat: follow the "Rest Mandate."

2. Strength/Resistance Training

Between your high-intensity workout days, you should do resistance training (strength training) to build muscle. Why?

First, muscle burns 4x more calories than fat. So the more muscle you have, the higher your base metabolism will be and the more calories you'll burn, even at rest. Muscle = great!

The second reason is even more important. Whenever you lose weight, you lose some muscle along with the fat. If you don't do strength training, up to 30% of the weight you lose can come from muscle loss. Muscle loss = bad = injuries.

Third, great muscle strength and tone are essential for functional living and health. Likewise, strength training helps preserve bone density, posture and balance.

So how do you get the most from strength training?

Here's the best way to train each muscle group at least once a week. Train them in zones for just 20 minutes per workout, at least once a week (see below). For example, one day you can work your upper body and then a couple of days later, train your lower body. You can also alternate between the front and back of your body.

And here comes another time where my advice is a little different than what you commonly hear. You see, most trainers tell you to rest between sets, but not me. *I want you to lift your weights or use resistance bands without resting between sets.* This method meets both cardio and strength requirements because you keep your heart rate elevated throughout your workout, increasing the amount of calories you burn per session. Your muscles will get tired as you go – just keep going and simply reduce the weight or repetitions accordingly so you'll complete the set.

Let me be clear – if you need to rest, of course you should. Listen to your body and start to gradually lessen the rest time.

When we talk about specific resistant training moves, I strongly suggest doing functional exercises – exercises that mimic activities of daily living. I am talking about pulling, pushing, jumping and squatting. They help move and strengthen your body so that it can perform the tasks you demand of it efficiently during your daily life. Remember my story about picking vegetables with my mom? Back then, I was working out in the gym regularly but was unable to do an ordinary task without getting out of breath. If you do functional exercises you will both strengthen your body and increase your ability to do what you need to do in your every day.

Basic functional exercises include:

- Squats
- Lunges
- Push-ups
- Crunches
- Military press: Hold a set of weights in your hands just above your shoulders close to your head. Push the weights up and lower them down to shoulder level. Repeat.
- Kettle bell swings (CAUTION: Please get an instructor to show you how to use kettle bells correctly. This is an

advanced activity, and as with all exercise, detailed attention to form is essential in order to receive the benefit of exercise while avoiding injury.)

- Bear crawl forwards and backwards

The bear crawl is one of my favorite exercises: I just love it! Like the kettle bell swings, it is a full body workout. Many of the world's top golfers use bear crawling to warm up, add strength and improve their coordination. What I love most about this move is that it takes you back to our most basic and primitive form of moving – crawling. Although basic in its appearance, crawling has magic in its innocence. It strengthens the arms and legs, and develops balance and coordination of arms, legs, neck and eyes. If you only had 10 minutes for exercise, forward and backward bear crawls will absolutely kick your butt and burn a ton of calories. Again, get a professional to show you exactly how to do this and please get clearance from your doctor before starting, especially if you have, or have had, any joint problems. This is book on health advice, not an exercise instruction manual. As always, I cannot overemphasize the importance of doing this exercise with correct form to avoid injury.

A professional demonstration of all these exercises is available on my website www.DrAraOnCall.com.

To maximize your workout, combine moves.

For example, I do squats and overhead military push-ups using 20-pound dumbbells. It kills after 10 reps. Or, try combining triceps extension with lunges.

Also be sure to avoid these common strength-training mistakes that lead to injury:

- Skipping warm-up: This can lead to sprains and tears.
- Sloppy form: As I've explained, proper form is the single most important factor in preventing injury. Stand straight, look forward, keep abs tight, and keep your knees positioned over the second toe of each foot.
- Stressing shoulders: Don't allow your elbows to extend more than two inches behind your body. Otherwise, you can overstretch the connective tissue in the front of the joints.
- Neglecting opposing muscle groups: In other words – if you work the front, work the back. It's the same premise with upper and lower body.

3. Core Exercises

This group of exercises provides the foundation for movement throughout your entire body. Exercises include crunches (aka sit-ups), planks, side planks and bridges.

By strengthening your core muscles (your torso/abdominal area and back), you help protect and support your back, make your spine and body less prone to injury, and gain greater balance and stability.

Your core muscles need at least two days of rest to recover, repair and rebuild, so really all you need to do is 10 minutes of crunches (aka sit-ups), planks, side planks and bridges once a week.

IMPORTANT! If you're new to exercising, find someone to teach you how to perform these important moves. They are the best investment for your body. Do them correctly and you won't strain your back.

A professional demonstration of all these exercises is available on my website www.DrAraOnCall.com.

4. Stretching

What do you notice as humans get older? They hunch, or stoop over. Their shoulders get curved forward and their knees don't straighten out. They hunch more. Their belly protrudes. And the vicious cycle continues.

One way you can avoid this is through daily stretching of four key areas. Stretch the front of your hips (hip extensors), hamstrings, pectoral area (front of the chest and shoulders) and lower back. Stretching improves circulation and increases the elasticity of muscle joints.

One way of stretching is by doing five basic yoga poses – Sun Salutation, Warrior One and Two, Downward Dog and Upward Dog.

If you're not sure how to do these stretches, please get a yoga instructor to show you.

Your MAGIC EXERCISE FORMULA

This is my exercise schedule for your optimal health:

- Three days of 20-minute high-intensity interval training (HIIT) with one full day between each session.
- One day of 20-minute resistance exercises/weight lifting.
- One day of 10-minute core exercises crunches/sit-ups, planks, side planks and bridges.
- Daily stretching of the hips, hamstrings, pectoral area and lower back as you cool down.

Let's put this into a daily plan/schedule you can easily follow for the rest of your life.

At a bare minimum, here's what you should do each week:

Monday, Wednesday and Friday: HIIT + Stretching as part of cool down

Tuesday: Resistance exercises + Stretching

Thursday: Core exercises + Stretching

If you have more time and as you get stronger, try this schedule:

Monday, Wednesday and Friday: HIIT + Stretching as part of cool down

Tuesday and Thursday: Core exercises + Resistance exercises + Stretching

NEVER – I mean NEVER – combine HIIT with resistance training or you'll send your Cortisol through the roof. And by now you know that Cortisol that is elevated beyond a certain point is detrimental to your health.

Hey, did you notice something? You have two days off! Awesome, right? Pick whatever days are most convenient for you! Remember, if you absolutely cannot squeeze a session in, do the four-minute Twenty Tens or bear crawl forwards and backwards twice at the very least.

Now if you have more time and you feel compelled to do some additional exercise, I highly recommend a slower paced long-distance run, the elliptical machine or a bike ride once a week. This longer duration exercise causes a release of endorphins that make you feel great! But based on current research, I wouldn't recommend more than 90 minutes of long-distance training more than once a week.

To wrap up the exercise component of your healthy new lifestyle, I'd like to address a few common questions I get from my clients.

Q: Why do you recommend lifting weights if I'm trying to lose fat? I don't want to look like a bodybuilder.

There's a risk of "bulking up" if ALL you do is weight training. But my Cortisol-balanced exercise regimen is a four-pronged approach with high-intensity cardio, core training and stretching mixed in as well. By blending cardio and strength training on different areas of the body, you'll lose inches all over. You'll also lengthen the muscles if you cross train, which slims you down everywhere.

Q: Is it possible to reach a plateau before I'm at my ideal weight? If so, how do I jump start my weight loss again?

If you've been exercising and cutting calories for several weeks, and you're no longer seeing or feeling the dramatic changes that you experienced in the early part of your training, you've probably hit a plateau. This typically occurs between weeks four and six. Do not be discouraged. This is great news. It occurs because your body has adapted to the new movements and nutrient supply. It's letting you know "I'm ready to be challenged again!"

When this happens, you break the plateau by revisiting and modifying our basic principles:

- Eat the right nutrients at the right time. Get stricter about avoiding processed foods or drinks and make sure you eat protein in the morning. Change up your food source; for example, swap celery sticks for raw almonds or eat more organic wild fish instead of beef.

Abs are made in the kitchen

Make sure you follow the strict rest mandates. If your body feels tired, it will slow down and this will show up as a reduction in your progress. Remember, do not perform High-Intensity Training on consecutive days. Professional endurance athletes often strategically schedule a week off from heavy training close to a major competition to rest their bodies, so that they can hit a new peak in time for the competition. So should you.

- Add variety to your workout. Your body is very smart. It will figure how to perform a new movement efficiently if you do it often. At that point, your progress slows down. You can kick-start your growth by adding more resistance, cranking up intensity or starting a completely new routine. I love trying a new routine because it keeps you mentally fresh and engaged. For example, swap lunges for step-ups.

Congratulations! You got this far... so you know how to exercise. Exercise is the gift that keeps on giving. Now let's learn about another gift... sleep!

CHAPTER 5

SLEEP FOR SUCCESS!

Sleep is extremely important to me. I need to rest and recover in order for the training I do to be absorbed by my body. Sleep is half my training

- Usain Bolt, the world's fastest man.

Why should you prioritize sleep when finding the time in your schedule feels impossible?

So many reasons!

Sleep rejuvenates the body and helps it make repairs. It's the calming function to keep Cortisol in balance. Sleep is also important in developing lean muscle tissue. When you work out, you're actually tearing your muscle. Sleep and proper nutrients help rebuild it.

On the other hand, the effects of long-term sleep deprivation are severe. Without enough sleep the body's immune system misfires, signs of aging appear rapidly and your body breaks down prematurely. You soon develop unwanted lines and wrinkles.

Chronic sleep deprivation also increases your body fat. Why? The latest research shows that participants with little sleep had reduced Leptin, which burns body fat, and elevated Ghrelin, which increases appetite. It also decreases the levels of the hormone that signals your brain when your body doesn't require any more food, so you overeat. So you end with a catastrophic combination of feeling hungry all the time, overeating but burning less body fat. This is compounded by the emotional comfort that eating provides when you are chronically tired. Alarmingly, overeating due to fatigue doesn't just happen to adults; it affects children too, leading to catastrophic childhood obesity.

In fact, if you're sleep-deprived, you're likely to have higher concentrations of sugar in your blood, which could contribute to development of a pre-diabetic condition. You are also more likely to have high blood pressure, heart disease and sleep apnea (short periods of not breathing at all). Perpetual sleepiness and fatigue also reduces the quality and quantity of your work.

Lack of sleep wrinkles the soul

You've been reading along seriously... so you must know that I am about to revisit the connection between Cortisol and sleep. Here's the bottom line: Poor sleep elevates Cortisol. Too much Cortisol keeps you awake. So you sleep less and a self-perpetuating cycle develops.

Lack of sleep is a serious problem. The nightly sleep for the average American has dropped from 10 hours (before the invention of the light bulb) to 6.9 hours, with a third of adults now getting even less than that. Lack of sleep is a national epidemic. According to the Centers for Disease Control and Prevention, insomnia plagues 50-70 million Americans each year and affects one in three adults, globally, with women and the elderly being the most susceptible.

I'll admit, for years, I took pride in functioning "perfectly well" on four hours of sleep. It was a rite of passage as part of my critical care, emergency medicine and surgical training. You had to prove you could function through significant sleep deprivation.

Why? I have no idea. I'd certainly want the most well-rested person looking after me if I was ever in the Intensive Care Unit, ER or operating room. Even after residency, I continued pushing myself to function on little sleep... I was exercising on my days off and not sleeping. In the long run, I was speeding down the highway to self-destruction. Is it any wonder I craved sugars and could never lose the excess belly fat? It was only when I came across the Sumo/Cortisol secret that I realized I needed to get serious about sleep right away.

I don't want you to make the same mistake I made.

But that's not all – sleep is not just about quantity. It's about quality too.

Let's indulge in some Snooze Science...

In 1937, Alfred Lee Loomis, an esteemed scientist, described two states of sleep: non-rapid eye movement (NREM) sleep and rapid eye movement (REM) sleep, where dreaming occurs. During sleep, the body cycles between non-REM and REM sleep.

NREM sleep is made up of Stages 1-4 (S1-S4).

Here is what occurs in each stage:

- Stage 1 – Transition to sleep – you are easily awakened here.
- Stage 2 – Light sleep
- Stage 3 and 4 – Deep sleep. You are difficult to wake and wake up groggy or disoriented. *Stages 3 and 4 are essential for well-being*. Here, every organ repairs, rejuvenates and recovers. Repair hormones are released. The immune system gets recharged and surveys for abnormal cells which could become cancerous. Most importantly, your mind rests in these stages so you wake up vibrant and refreshed.

A completed cycle of sleep consists of a progression from Stages 1-4 before REM sleep. We usually have four to five cycles in a typical seven- to eight-hour sleep period, and we spend varying amounts of time in each stage.

The quality of your sleep is directly proportional to the amount spent in Stage 3 and 4. As we get older, we sleep more lightly and get less Stage 3 and 4 sleep... and less time is spent repairing the body. This is one reason we start "getting old," breaking down more easily, becoming prone to cancers and taking longer to recover from simple illnesses like the common cold.

Most people don't realize that we can sleep without ever getting to the critical Stage 3-4 of sleep that our body needs to rejuvenate. I often see examples of this in my patients suffering from depression and I personally went through this after a painful breakup. I spent countless hours in bed asleep yet woke up feeling like I had hardly slept and experienced a profound loss of energy.

Most doctors who are on call overnight will tell you they don't feel well-rested the next day, even if they do not get called during the night. Subconsciously, their fear of sleeping through their pager keeps them from sleeping deeply and getting to stages 3-4.

On the other hand, can you recall a time when you slept for a much shorter time than you are used to and yet woke up refreshed? On those nights, you spent a more significant amount of your sleep in deep sleep.

It is a common experience that a problem difficult at night is resolved in the morning after the committee of sleep has worked on it.

- John Steinbeck

Insomnia is such an awful feeling that most people will resort to medication out of desperation. Today one in four of us use prescription sleeping aids. It may be necessary in some instances, but for most of my patients, addressing lifestyles, sleep hygiene, exercise and diet would improve the quantity and quality of their sleep. In my experience, sleep medications help get you to sleep but do not buy you the deep sleep your body requires to recover and feel fully rested.

But please, if you are already taking meds, don't just stop suddenly. I don't want you to suffer sudden withdrawal symptoms. Consider easing off slowly with the help of your doctor. You can make lifestyle changes to improve the quality and quantity of your sleep simultaneously. Remember:

Small Changes + Time = **Huge Results**

Finally – your Insider's Prescription to healthy, quality sleeping.

I understand how painful the struggle to sleep can be, but I want you to know that in many cases there are alternatives to pharmaceutical/medication. Changing sleep habits may be difficult at first, but if it means you sleep better, you will be glad you made the effort! Try implementing these recommendations...

- Make a routine at bedtime. Brush your teeth, wash your face and calm your mind.
- As I said before, avoid stimulation at least three hours before bed, including coffee, eating and exercise – unless it's a healthy romantic encounter, which is good for you. (Studies show that people who have strong romantic relationships and frequent sex live longer. Awesome!!)
- Avoid electromagnetic fields (EMF) close to your bed – they play a big role in poor sleep and Cortisol spikes. EMF are produced by electronic devices. Try to remove

cordless phones, cell phones, laptops and even televisions from the bedroom. At a bare minimum, move alarm clocks and other electrical devices away from your head. If these devices must be used, keep them as far away from your bed as possible, preferably at least three feet.

- Also try to turn off electronics at least 90 minutes before bedtime. Electronic reading devices trigger Cortisol release due to the light they emit. Your brain perceives the light as being daytime and releases Cortisol instead of sleep hormones (Melatonin), which interferes with sleep cycles. Stick with printed material in bed.

- Create a soothing sleeping environment. Cover your windows with blackout shades or heavy drapes. Close your bedroom door, get rid of night-lights and refrain from turning on any light during the night, even when getting up to go to the bathroom. If you're traveling, do everything you can to mimic your home environment. Try using a mask.

- Don't drink alcohol to get drowsy. It will cause your blood sugar to yo-yo through the night. This triggers an unwanted release of Cortisol in the middle of the night and leads to poor sleep.

- Use sleep medications as a last resort. Of course, we all go through extremely stressful periods when worry, anxiety, grief or loss keep us awake. Your doctor will guide you, based on your circumstances, if you need to go on a short course of sleeping medication. In those situations, sleep medications are your temporary friends while you ride out the storm. However, as a long-term solution – they're not your friends! They don't get you to stage 4 of sleep, and this impairs your Cortisol balance. Aside from being ineffective in helping you get to deep sleep, sleeping pills also come with a slew of detrimental and potentially dangerous side effects. For starters, they can be addictive, which means that when you want to stop taking them, you'll likely suffer withdrawal symptoms perhaps worse than your initial insomnia. Other common side effects include weight gain, sleepwalking and eating in your sleep. You're also more apt to get into a traffic accident if you are using sleeping pills. (Ambien ranks among the top 10 drugs found in the bloodstreams of impaired drivers, according to some state toxicology labs.)

Again, do not simply stop taking sleeping pills if you are using them. Consult your doctor. If appropriate, you will need to wean off them slowly.

Even if you're a shift worker or if you're someone who can't escape a variable schedule, you can still practice good sleep hygiene. Though I do varying shifts in the ER, I work hard to create a sleep environment and routine that is conducive to quality sleep. There is not a one size fits all approach. I had to find what worked for me – and you do too.

Take a rest. A field that has rested gives bountiful crops

- Ovid

Here's another approach you could try. You may be able to overcome an inadequate night's sleep by scheduling in a short nap in the day. I'm not talking about two- or three-hour snoozes which sometimes occur in front of the TV on a weekend. I am talking about a 15- to 20-minute power nap.

Power naps recharge the brain without letting you enter an actual sleep cycle. This is why you awake refreshed and sharp as a tack. They also lower your blood pressure. You may also notice that you have improved circulation, muscles are more relaxed and joints are less stiff after a brief rest period.

Additionally, a short nap is a major form of stress reduction because it releases the repair hormones that balance out Cortisol and also reduce inflammation and "stress."

So, what do you do if you practice everything that I suggested and you still struggle with getting enough quality sleep? It's time for the four slumber seducers – exercise, limiting Melatonin drainers, Feng Shui and reducing stress.

First, exercise!

If you follow Your MAGIC EXERCISE FORMULA in this guide, you'll enjoy better sleep and more energy. And... healthy sleep is every bit as valuable to your overall well-being as exercise and good nutrition.

Here's how exercise helps you sleep better:

- Working out regularly has been shown to reduce episodes of insomnia. Vigorous exercise during the day (not in the evening!) helps you fall asleep AND stay asleep more easily.

Adults who exercised 20 to 30 minutes every other day in the early afternoon found that their required time to fall asleep was reduced by half and total sleep time increased by almost an hour.

- Exercise increases the time you spend in the deepest sleep phase (Stages 3 and 4).
- Exercise supports improved sleep quality by producing smoother, more regular transitions between the cycles and phases of sleep.

I hope by now I've convinced you to exercise. Next, you need to limit what I call Melatonin drainers.

What's Melatonin? Melatonin is a hormone produced by a pea-sized gland in the middle of your brain called the pineal gland, which is affected by light and dark. At night, when it gets dark, your pineal gland switches "on" and begins producing Melatonin to be released into your blood, which makes you feel sleepy.

When functioning normally, your Melatonin levels will stay elevated for about 12 hours (usually between 9 p.m. and 9 a.m.). Then, as the sun rises, your pineal gland turns "off" and the Melatonin levels in your blood decrease.

Ideally and under normal conditions, your sleepiness should gradually increase throughout the day, peaking just before you go to bed at night.

There are three main Melatonin drainers that keep us from sleeping well – light and electromagnetic radiation, noise and temperature, all of which spike our Cortisol at the inappropriate time.

Drainer 1: Light and electromagnetic radiation

This little gland is very sensitive to light and dark. That explains why light-emitting electronic gadgets should be avoided before going to bed and why something as simple as turning on a light in the middle of the night can interfere with your sleep.

Also be aware of what's on the other side of your bedroom wall and under the floor. In other words, avoid sleeping with your head against a wall that has electric meters, circuit breaker panels, televisions or stereos, for example, on the other side. All of these are sources of magnetic fields that you should sleep at least four feet away from to limit exposure during sleep. If you have to leave a light on, install so-called "low blue" light bulbs in your bedroom and bathroom. These emit an amber light that will not suppress Melatonin production.

Drainer 2: Noise

In order to get a good night's sleep, you want your sleepiness level to be high, and the noise

level to be low. If noise is greater than your level of sleepiness, you will not fall asleep.

Noise can include any *kind of stimulation that inhibits or disrupts sleep* – not just traditional

sound — and is generally classified into three types:

- Mind: The most common type is referred to as "cognitive popcorn," or unstoppable thoughts running through your mind at night.
- Body: Physical pain, discomfort, indigestion, and side

effects from prescription drugs or residual caffeine from drinking coffee too late in the day can be a major problem when you're trying to fall asleep.

- Environmental: Environmental noise is usually obvious, such as noises in your room or house, a snoring partner, music or lights.

Often the reason why people can't fall asleep is not because of a lack of sleepiness, but rather because of excessive noise.

Drainer 3: Temperature

Make sure your bedroom's temperature promotes sound sleep: Although there is a wide range of individual preferences, research suggests a temperature from 60 to 68 degrees F (15.5 to 20 C) is the most beneficial for sleep. A hotter or cooler room can lead to restless sleep.

Address those three Melatonin drainers and you will almost immediately notice a difference in the quality of your sleep... There's more to sleep than you thought – right? Stick with me.

After getting your exercise and limiting your Melatonin drainers... it's time to try Feng Shui.

Feng Shui, which originates in the Chinese philosophy of Taoism, instructs us on how to arrange rooms, furniture, offices, houses and other living spaces to maximize a favorable energy flow.

Basically, when your sleep area is cluttered or poorly arranged, so is your subconscious mind… and deep sleep is less likely. In short, unclutter and clean up your bedroom. It works.

Here are additional Feng Shui recommendations that may help promote relaxing sleep:

- Place your bed in the middle of a wall, away from sharp corners. Why? The energy tends to be stagnant (non-flowing) in corners. Plus, sharp edges of desks, bookcases and other furniture can also disturb positive energy and should be avoided if possible.

- Place your bed away from windows. It is believed that energy drains out the window, so putting your bed beneath or directly next to a window can drain your energy.

- Position your bed so the soles of your feet do not directly face the door when you are lying face-up in bed. Feng Shui masters believe that your energy will be pulled away from your feet in this position. Having said that, it's best to have a full view of anyone coming in the door. If you can't do this directly, hang a mirror to reflect the entranceway.

And now for the fourth and perhaps the most difficult sleep solution to tackle – reducing stress.

"But I can't chill out! I have deadlines, bills, things to do!" Yes, everyone does... but if you allow stress to rule your life, guess what? It *will* rule your life, and in the end it may actually end your life.

When you push your body and mind to the edge through overworking, poor diet, lack of exercise, lousy sleep and no relaxation or recovery, chances are you're miserable. Plus it's also pretty likely that you're unhealthy.

The bad news is *time flies.*
The good news is *you're the pilot.*

– Michael Altshuler

You DO have a choice in the matter.

If you're allowing stress to dominate your days, try these suggestions:

- If at all possible say no! Don't take the extra shift, don't volunteer for the program at school, just don't do whatever IT might be. Instead, go home and unplug for a few hours.
- Consider silencing the phone and not checking email on your days off even for an hour. Trust me, I know that for many of you, this is a big ask. Maybe you are a parent or your job requires that you are always reachable. Of course, you need to fulfill your responsibilities, but if possible, try to find ways to disengage from electronics. Try it for an hour and build on it. Everyone's situation is different, but the goal is to be totally present with those who you care about deeply. That requires switching off your distractors.
- Set a bedtime. Routines worked when you were a child and they'll do the same thing at this stage of your life.

- Learn to let off steam appropriately. I take out all my frustrations on little white golf balls or when I work out. And, trust me, those dearest to me can tell when I do and don't work out! I also talk to friends or my significant other about frustrations. You will be surprised by how helpful exercise and talking can be.

- Mentally check out. A few hours before you head to bed each day, make a conscious effort to forget everything. It gives the brain a bit of breathing room to do the tasks it needs to do in order to keep you healthy. Again, I know this may not be possible for many of you, but even five or 10 minutes are better than nothing. Journaling your thoughts works precisely for this reason. It's almost as if you have taken it out of your mind and transferred it to paper so your mind can disconnect and sleep. It empties out your mind and allows you to rest. You will even breathe easier. This is my go-to method when I get stressed or overwhelmed. This single act will add vibrant years to your life.

- Breathe consciously. I'm sure you have heard this before, but have you practiced it religiously? Deep and focused breathing is an optimal method of relaxing and inducing sleep. Before bedtime, sit upright with your hand on your abdomen and simply pay attention to your slow inhalation and exhalation. It's remarkably relaxing. Remember:

Small Changes + Time = **Huge Results**.

- Get a massage before aches and pains set in. Massage relaxes muscles, keeps joints supple and helps detoxify the body. Massage sounds like an indulgence, but it is actually an investment in longevity. It can, however, be expensive, so look for less expensive ways to get similar results. Scope out a credible local massage school where massages will be more reasonably priced. Take a massage class with your partner and trade massages on a regular basis. Here again, small changes equal big results. If you never get a massage, and all of a sudden you and your partner begin incorporating five minutes every week, it's an achievement! Another way to relax your muscles is to soak in Epsom salts and organic lavender oil before bed. Try this for seven consecutive days and I promise you will never look back.

- Learn a new skill. The two things that have consistently been shown to maintain cognition and a healthy brain are learning a musical instrument and learning a new language, but any new skill brings about a sense of wonder and challenge that is essential to feeling fully alive. When you feel alive, you are less stressed!

- Consider getting a pet, especially a cat or dog. Studies have shown that having pets reduces Cortisol and improves your mood and overall well-being. In fact, dogs are used to treat depression, anxiety and ADHD. Pets shower you with unconditional love. They listen to you vent. Petting them actually lowers your blood pressure and heart rate while playing and walking with them helps you move. Plus they help you socialize, which is a common quality of those who live beyond a hundred!

- Consider professional therapy. A good therapist is worth their weight in gold because they are trained to deal with emotions and feelings that you may not be able to handle on your own.

I know how hard this is. We have become so accustomed to fulfilling the never-ending demands and expectations of this world that stress is seen as the norm of everyday life. Even our vacations are stressful. Most of us feel like we need another vacation to recover from the last vacation. But, if you just accept it and don't try to change it, stress will shorten your life. When you think about the people depending on you, don't you want to take steps to lower your stress level today?

Who is counting on *you* to be the *healthiest*?

Finally, consider going herbal if my previous ideas are not helping. There are a variety of herbs that can help you fall asleep and stay asleep.

These are my favorites:

Valerian: We think valerian increases the levels of the brain's calming neurotransmitter GABA. It's commonly found in most sleep-time tea blends. You can either drink the tea version or you can take 400-900 mg of capsules an hour before bedtime. It takes about two to three weeks to work and it shouldn't be used for more than one month at a time.

Melatonin: Melatonin is a popular remedy to help people fall asleep when the sleep/wake cycle has been disturbed, such as shift workers or people with jet lag. Taking 1-3 mg is safe, although fatigue and depression have occasionally been reported with use.

Lavender: Use this essential oil in a bath or put a few drops under your pillow.

Magnesium: Magnesium is a natural sedative. Deficiency of magnesium can result in difficulty sleeping, as well as constipation, muscle tremors or cramps, anxiety, irritability and pain. While you can get sufficient magnesium from your diet (legumes and seeds, dark leafy green vegetables, almonds, cashews), for insomnia, it's easier to take tablets. The standard magnesium dosage for adults is 280-300 mg per day for most women and 270-400 mg per day for men.

IMPORTANT: Sleep disturbances could be a primary medical condition due to sleep apnea, thyroid disorders, depression, anxiety, uncontrolled blood pressure and certain tumors. If this sounds like you or you cannot sleep soundly after trying the above, see a doctor to make sure you don't have a serious medical condition.

A final note on sleep: Sleep and rest are two different things – and you need *both*.

For instance, I discourage you from watching TV or reading if you're having a hard time getting to sleep... but if you're not able to stop yourself from thinking too much, you have to find a way to rest. In this case, sitting and watching TV, playing a board game with the kids, reading a good book or learning a new skill are all good ways to keep your mind off your work, obligations, the endless to-do list and the stuff that packs your daily life and creates difficulty with sleep or relaxation.

Remember that the Sabbath day was created because even GOD rested on the seventh day. If the maker of all things can check out for a full day... it's safe to say that the world won't really notice if you do the same. A full day may not always be realistic, but seek out pockets of time where you can. Remember, your body and mind will notice if you refuse to relax and recover, and it will actually weaken your work and life performance.

You have now learned that improving the quality of your sleep can be done by making long-lasting lifestyle modifications.

By following the advice in this section, I hope you can get your body (and maybe even your household) on a deep sleep schedule that produces mental clarity, loads of energy and productive days!

Here's a recap on how to get the best sleep of your life... for the rest of your life.

- Avoid eating, caffeine, alcohol and exercising at least three hours before bedtime.
- Turn off any electronics near your bed. Or better yet, remove them from the bedroom.
- Create a "sleep sanctuary" with darkness and a cool temperature.
- Try our many stress-reducing techniques to prepare for a

good night's sleep, especially journaling.

- Set a regular bedtime and try to get seven to eight hours of sleep every night.
- Avoid turning on lights during the night, even if you get up for a bathroom visit – this will interrupt your deep sleep. Use a blue light.
- If you're still struggling to fall asleep or stay asleep, consider checking out the herbal suggestions.

Now you have the keys to quality food, hydration, exercise and sleep. In the next chapter, you'll put it all together for a healthy, happy, Cortisol-balanced life!

CHAPTER 6

CRUSH IT! IT'S TIME TO TURBOCHARGE YOUR LIFE NOW!

Life is not a brief candle. It is a splendid torch that must be made to burn as brightly as possible before it is handed on to the next generation.

- George Bernard Shaw

You cannot change the past, but you can create your future. So make it magnificent and take your life to another level. It's never too late to become what you might have been.

It's time to crush it!

With everything I've shown you... you're ready to take your first steps.

But please... take baby steps, make small changes, bite off small chunks and give yourself plenty of time.

Strive for *progress* not *perfection*

Why? It's not uncommon for drastic and enormous bites to lead to indigestion in the form of failure, turmoil and a huge sense of frustration. Similarly, weight gain does not happen overnight and neither does weight loss.

Instead, take some time now to understand what you need to do in order to get a slimmer, sexier, healthier body that serves you well for many years to come.

Here's a reminder of the 10 main points I've covered in this guide:

1. Assess your nutritional choices and level of fitness.

2. Write down clear, specific goals with timelines to keep on track.

3. Ask yourself "why" and answer honestly.

4. Use the information in Chapter 2 to follow your FUELING FORMULA.

Remember the five fundamentals:
- Eat the best foods for your body.
- Eat slowly.
- Eat only until you're almost full.

- Eat three medium meals and three snacks.
- Half your body weight in pounds = ounces of fluids you require a day to stay hydrated.

5. Now create an exercise plan based on the MAGIC EXERCISE FORMULA in Chapter 4 and make it a top priority! At a bare minimum, follow this easy plan each week:

- Monday, Wednesday and Friday: HIIT + Stretching as part of cool down
- Tuesday: Resistance exercises + Stretching
- Thursday: Core exercises + Stretching
- Saturday and Sunday: Have fun with light exercise or none at all! (off days are your choice)

Remember: Three days a week of High-Intensity Interval Training is all you need each week, with rest days in between! It's 20 minutes at a time. Please try to fit this in. It's an investment in your future health.

6. Assess the quality of your sleep... honestly.

7. Make a plan to implement the changes identified in Chapter 5 as needed to improve your quality of sleep and try to find more time for Cortisol-balanced slumber.

8. Mandate relaxation and restful times that include "checking out" from stress.

9. Keep a journal to help you navigate difficult and unchangeable relationships at work or   home.

10. Stick with your plan and track your progress to make sure you're meeting your short, mid- and long-term goals for Cortisol balance and feeling great around the clock.

That's it. That's the simple Insider's Prescription to Turbocharge Your Life Now

—your keys to losing weight and feeling great forever.

Eat well, move daily, hydrate often, sleep lots, love your body. *Repeat.*

I remember the day I deciphered the Sumo hieroglyphic. I got scared. As much as I respected my big friends in Japan, I didn't want to die prematurely like they do.

I thought of all the days I spent sitting in front of the TV with pizza, chicken wings and wine. Or the days when it was so busy in the ER, I literally went 14 hours without eating and then wolfed down my favorite Chinese takeout.

But I was not informed. And now I am… just like you!

Apply the principles in this book and you will transform your life. Start right now even if you feel like you are not ready. If we wait for the moment when everything, absolutely everything, is right, we shall never begin. Whatever you can do, or dream you can do, begin it. Boldness has genius, power and magic in it.

As you finish this book and start your journey to better health, let's go back to PGA Physical Therapist Marc Wahl who wrote the introduction to this book.

Six years ago, Marc asked me out of the blue, "What do you think of this medication called methotrexate?" I told him the pros and cons and then I asked him why he wanted to know. He told me that his psoriasis was out of control. He had had blood tests done and had abnormal results, pointing towards a rheumatological disorder. His doctor advised him to start taking this medication. Marc's a very smart guy – he knew the medication had serious side effects.

I joined him on a walk on the course, following one of our players. I questioned him about his lifestyle; asking about his diet, sleep, exercise, what he ate and drank, all in minute detail. He told me about his psoriasis, joint pain, fatigue and generally feeling out of shape. Despite an amazing career on the PGA tour as a highly sought-after physical therapist, he himself was in poor health.

It became increasingly obvious to me that he was a victim of excess Cortisol.

First, he was working very long hours. He started at 5 a.m. on most days and sometimes his last client was at 10 p.m. His work was labor intensive: Physical therapy is strenuous work and he was working hard for long periods with no fuel.

Regularly he'd go for 10-12 hours without eating. He was slim, but his eyes lacked sparkle.

When he did eat at the end of the day, he ate very quickly and drank too much alcohol, before hitting the bed in a heap of exhaustion. On a good night, he got six hours of sleep.

This cycle would repeat itself day after day for weeks on end.

On top of all this, he felt stressed and guilty because he was spending so much time away from family. When he was home, he made up for this by being super dad and husband leaving little time for his personal rest or recovery. His path to self-destruction was fully ablaze, fueled by unbalanced Cortisol.

If it doesn't *challenge you,* it doesn't *change you*

– Fred DeVito

Because he was motivated to feel better and avoid medication, I got him to agree to a few simple lifestyle modifications he could make immediately:

- Eat breakfast and eat at least three meals a day based on his body weight and calorie intake.
- Drink water equaling half his body weight in ounces.
- Promise to cut back his alcohol intake to one drink per night.
- Undertaking no additional exercise because his physical therapy work was like a HIIT session multiple times a day.

Plus, through his own initiative, he bought an audiobook by Eckhart Tolle that he could listen to during any downtime throughout the day, to reduce stress and help him stay in the present.

I kept tabs on his progress over the next few months. He seemed to be doing fine. Six months went by before we met at another tournament. He was doing more than fine – he looked like a magnificent Viking! I was greeted by a huge hug and smile after which he proceeded to pick me up over his shoulders, laughing, "I feel incredible bro!"

Small Changes + Time = **Huge Results**

There was life in his eyes. He had a youthful complexion. His muscles were rippling. He looked strong and powerful. His psoriasis and joint pain were completely gone. His blood levels were nearly back to normal. Without any medication. All in six months.

Soon, everyone around him started commenting on how good he looked. That gave him more incentive to become even more vigilant about what he ate and drank.

Sure, Marc still had some sleep deprivation because of the demanding nature of his work. And he could not ease up on his physically taxing job. But he still experienced a huge improvement in how good he felt and looked. How? By following the Cortisol-balanced diet, squeezing in naps and making simple lifestyle modifications 80% of the time, he got away with the other 20%.

Mark is 47 and he now looks and performs like he is 30! He's better at his job and he functions better with his family, especially with his kids.

Marc started my program at age 43. He was working full-time, with abnormal blood tests, a hectic travel schedule, a young family and celebrity clients that he cared about immensely. If he can make these changes you can do it too!

Of this I am certain: the human body is extremely forgiving. Any damage you've done to your body can be reversed for the most part. Remember those *Biggest Loser* contestants who beat diabetes? And even if you're not suffering from disease... keep in mind that a lack of disease does not equal health, as I've explained.

When life isn't fair, *change the rules*

If you follow the MAGIC FORMULAS in this book, at least 80% of the time – you WILL lose weight, enjoy more energy, sleep better and add vibrant, energetic years to your life. You can indulge within reason the other 20% of time... your body will forgive you.

So start today and never look back. Follows these four tips for success:

- Take small bites at each of these changes and soon you'll be forming great habits.
- Expect to fail sometimes, but NEVER GIVE UP!
- Don't expect instant results, but be prepared for a kick-ass reaction when someone sees you for the first time in weeks.
- Do not try any other diet or system for at least six months. This gives The Insider's Prescription a chance to make a

meaningful difference.

In fact, I'm including a Turbocharge Your Life Contract for you at the end of this chapter. Sign it, print a copy and hang it on your refrigerator for daily inspiration. Commit to this system in writing, and declare it to your family and friends!

The body *achieves* what the mind *believes*.

Next, take four photos of yourself. Three should be full body. Take one from the front, one from the side and one from the back. Then take one from the front that's from the shoulders up. I want you to have a record of your starting point so you can look back later and take pride in how far you've come.

Then, find a picture of someone whose physique you admire and put their picture next to yours, but do not include their face. Just their body. This is key, because I want you to focus on their physique (I used a neck down picture of Mark Wahlberg! The pictures and contract were on my fridge door reminding me every day). And amazing things will happen. The photos of you and your role model will become embedded in your subconscious and slowly you will start to make changes that get you closer to your goals. You become what your mind focuses on. This is a tangible way to motivate yourself. Then take new photos every six weeks and replace the old. Document your journey in writing and on video – this will serve as a constant reminder of how hard you worked and why you want to keep it up! Also, please send your pictures and video to me at www.DRARAONCALL.COM. I can't wait to see your transformation. You could become a featured role model on my site.

What you do *today*
can improve all your *tomorrows*

You cannot change your past but you can shape your future. Consciously focusing on a healthy body is the first step in your new life. Be the commander that your family and friends are looking for. Be powerful beyond measure.

I'll leave you with the most important lesson working in the ER teaches me every day:

Tomorrow is never promised. Make every day count.

Till our paths meet, enjoy the journey and above all, live life on your terms.

TURBOCHARGE MY LIFE NOW

I, _____ will ONLY follow the MAGIC FORMULAS for eating, drinking, exercising and sleeping for the next six months. I will not be distracted by "quick fix" or fad diets, so-called instant remedies or infomercial gizmos that promise results without much effort which seduced me in the past.

IT'S MY TIME TO SHINE.
I CHOOSE TO LEAD NOT FOLLOW.
I WILL BELIEVE NOT DOUBT.
I AM POWERFUL BEYOND MEASURE.
I LIVE ON MY TERMS.

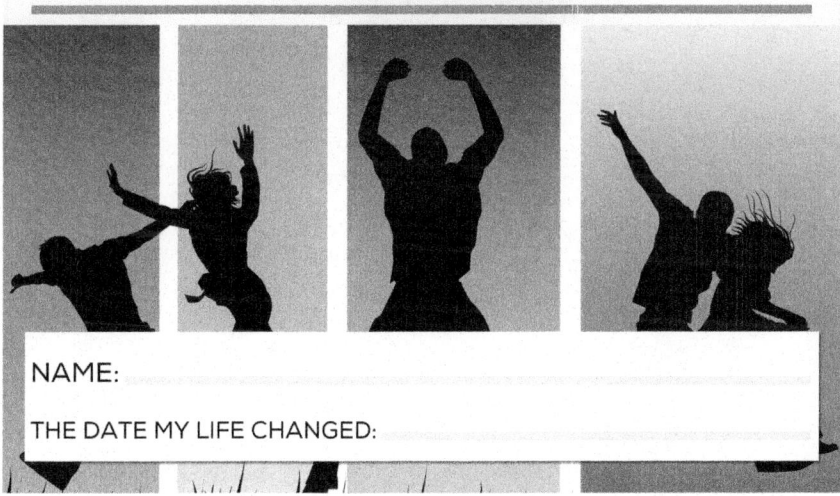

NAME: _____

THE DATE MY LIFE CHANGED: _____

ABOUT THE AUTHOR

A lifelong athlete, Dr. Ara Suppiah knows what it takes for anyone to achieve his or her peak potential, and thrives on creating optimal health in each of his patients. After 18 years of practicing medicine around the world, he has a reputation for getting quick results and communicating in a simple manner that resonates with patients from all walks of life.

Dr. Ara is a practicing ER physician, Chief Wellness Officer for Florida Emergency Physicians and an Assistant Professor at the University of Central Florida Medical School. He is a highly sought after personal physician for the PGA Tour of America, treating an A-list roster that includes 2013 U.S. Open Champion Justin Rose, Ian Poulter, Steve Stricker, Gary Woodland, Henrik Stenson, Hunter Mahan, J.B. Holmes and Golf Hall of Fame member Vijay Singh. Earlier in his career, Dr. Ara was a physician on the European Tour and the European Ryder Cup Teams.

He's been featured in the BBC series *Trauma* and is the creator of Golf Medicine and High Performance Medicine at www. TourCouncil.com. For more information on Dr. Ara Suppiah and his services which include life changing keynote speeches, corporate training and seminars, please visit www.DrAraOnCall.com

REFERENCES

John K. Francis. Coffea arabica L. RUBIACEAE. Factsheet of U.S. Department of Agriculture, Forest Service.

Freedman N, et al. Association of Coffee Drinking with Total and Cause-Specific Mortality. N Engl J Med 2012; 366:1891-1904

Hamza TH, et al. Genome-wide gene-environment study identifies glutamate receptor gene GRIN2A as a Parkinson's disease modifier gene via interaction with coffee. PLoS Genet. 2011 Aug 7(8):e1002237.

Gavrieli A, et al. Caffeinated coffee does not acutely affect energy intake, appetite, or inflammation but prevents serum Cortisol concentrations from falling in healthy men. J Nutr. 2011 Apr 1;141(4):703-7.

Andrade AM, Greene GW, Melanson KJ.J Eating slowly led to decreases in energy intake within

meals in healthy women. Am Diet Assoc. 2008 Jul;108(7):1186-91. doi:

10.1016/j.jada.2008.04.026.   http://www.ncbi.nlm.nih.gov/pubmed/18589027

Cornelis MC, et al. Coffee, CYP1A2 Genotype, and Risk of Myocardial Infarction. JAMA. 2006; 295(10):1135-1141

Wisborg K, et al. Maternal consumption of coffee during pregnancy and stillbirth and infant death in first year of life: prospective study. BMJ. 2003 326 (7386): 420.

Richelle M, et al. Comparison of the Antioxidant Activity of Commonly Consumed Polyphenolic Beverages (Coffee, Cocoa, and Tea) Prepared per Cup Serving. J. Agric. Food Chem., 2001, 49 (7), pp 3438–3442

Leitzmann MF, et al. A prospective study of coffee consumption and the risk of symptomatic gallstone disease in men. JAMA. 1999 281:2106-12

Leitzmann MF, et al. Coffee intake is associated with lower risk of symptomatic gallstone disease in women. Gastroenterology. 2002 Dec; 123(6):1823-30

Webster Ross G, et al. Association of Coffee and Caffeine Intake With the Risk of Parkinson Disease. JAMA. May 24, 2000, 283:20

Hancock DB, et al. Smoking, Caffeine, and Nonsteroidal Anti-inflammatory Drugs in Families With Parkinson Disease. Arch Neurol. 2007; 64(4):576-580.

Klatsky AL, et al. Coffee, Cirrhosis, and Transaminase Enzymes. Arch Intern Med. 2006; 166:1190-1195.

van Dam RM, Hu FB. Coffee consumption and risk of type 2 diabetes: a systematic review. JAMA. 2005 Jul 6; 294(1):97-104.

Tavani, A, et al. Coffee and tea intake and risk of oral, pharyngeal and esophageal cancer. Oral Oncol. 2003 39(7): 695-700.

Ganmaa D, Willett WC, Li TY, et al. Coffee, tea, caffeine and risk of breast cancer: a 22-year follow-up. Int J Cancer 2008 122(9): 2071-6.

Inoue M, Yoshimi I, Sobue T, Tsugane S. Influence of Coffee Drinking on Subsequent Risk of Hepatocellular Carcinoma: A Prospective Study in Japan. JNCI Journal of the National Cancer Institute 97 (4): 293-300

Nkondjock A. Coffee consumption and the risk of cancer: an overview. Cancer Lett. 2009 May 18; 277(2):121-5.

Arab L. Epidemiologic evidence on coffee and cancer. Nutr Cancer. 2010; 62(3):271-83.

Somoza V, et al. Activity-Guided Identification of a Chemopreventive Compound in Coffee Beverage Using in Vitro and in Vivo Techniques. J Agric Food Chem. 2003 51 (23), pp 6861–6869

American Association for Cancer Research Frontiers in Cancer Prevention Research Conference, Houston, Dec. 6-8, 2009.

Jarvis MJ. Does caffeine intake enhance absolute levels of cognitive performance? Psychopharmacology. 2 December 2005, 110:1-2, 45-52.

Johnson-Kozlow M, et al. Coffee Consumption and Cognitive Function among Older Adults. Am JEpidemiol 2002; 156:842-850

Lopez-Garcia E, et al. The Relationship of Coffee Consumption with Mortality. Annals of Internal Medicine 2008 Jun 17; 148(12):904-14.

Koizumi A, Mineharu Y, Wada Y, Iso H et al. Coffee, green tea, black tea and oolong tea consumption and risk of mortality from cardiovascular disease in Japanese men and women. Journal of Epidemiology and Community Health 2011 65: 230-240.

Armstrong LE. Caffeine, body fluid-electrolyte balance, and exercise performance. Int J Sport Nutr Exer Metab. 2002 Jun; 12(2):189-206.

Maughan RJ, Griffin J. Caffeine ingestion and fluid balance: a review. J Hum Nutr Diet. 2003 16(6):411–420.

Eskelinen MH, et al. Midlife Coffee and Tea Drinking and the

Risk of Late-Life Dementia: A Population-Based CAIDE Study. J Alzheimers Dis. January 2009. 16(1);85-91

Buscemi N, Vandermeer B, Hooton N, Pandya R, Tjosvold L, Hartling L, Vohra S, Klassen TP, Baker G. Efficacy and safety of exogenous melatonin for secondary sleep disorders and sleep disorders accompanying sleep restriction: meta-analysis. BMJ. 2006 Feb 18; 332(7538):385-93

Cao C, et al. Caffeine suppresses amyloid-beta levels in plasma and brain of Alzheimer's disease transgenic mice. J Alzheimers Dis. 2009; 17(3):681-97.

Mariangela Rondanelli, et al. The Effect of Melatonin, Magnesium and Zinc on Primary Insomnia in Long-Term Care Facility Residents in Italy: A Double-Blind, Placebo-Controlled Clinical Trial; Journal of the American Geriatrics Society. January 2011

André La Gerche, Andrew T. Burns, Don J. Mooney, Warrick J. Inder, Andrew J. Taylor, Jan Bogaert, Andrew I. MacIsaac, Hein Heidbüchel and David L. Prior. Exercise-induced right ventricular dysfunction and structural remodeling in endurance athletes. http://eurheartj.oxfordjournals.org/content/early/2011/12/05/eurheartj.ehr397.abstract

Tomas G. Neilan, MD; James L. Januzzi, MD; Elizabeth Lee-Lewandrowski, PhD; Thanh-Thao Ton-Nu, MD; Danita M. Yoerger, MD; Davinder S. Jassal, MD; Kent B. Lewandrowski, MD; Arthur

J. Siegel, MD; Jane E. Marshall, RDCS; Pamela S. Douglas, MD; David Lawlor, MD; Michael H. Picard, MD; Malissa J. Wood, MD. Myocardial Injury and Ventricular Dysfunction Related to Training Levels Among Nonelite Participants in the Boston Marathon. http:// circ.ahajournals.org/content/114/22/2325.abstract

Siegel AJ, Stec JJ, Lipinska I, Van Cott EM, Lewandrowski KB, Ridker PM, Tofler GH. Effect of marathon running on inflammatory and hemostatic markers. http://www.ncbi.nlm.nih. gov/pubmed/11676965

Wilson M, O'Hanlon R, Prasad S, Deighan A, Macmillan P, Oxborough D, Godfrey R, Smith G, Maceira A, Sharma S, George K, Whyte G.J. Diverse patterns of myocardial fibrosis in lifelong, veteran endurance athletes. Appl Physiol. 2011 Jun; 110(6):1622-6. doi: 10.1152/japplphysiol.01280.2010. Epub 2011 Feb 17.

Begoña Benito, MD*; Gemma Gay-Jordi, PhD*; Anna Serrano-Mollar, PhD; Eduard Guasch, MD; Yanfen Shi, MD; Jean-Claude Tardif, MD; Josep Brugada, MD, PhD; Stanley Nattel, MD†; Lluis Mont, MD, PhD. Cardiac Arrhythmogenic Remodeling in a Rat Model of Long-Term Intensive Exercise Training. http://circ. ahajournals.org/content/123/1/13.short

Mozaffarian D, Katan MB, Ascherio A, Stampfer MJ, Willett WC (2006). "Trans fatty acids and cardiovascular disease". *N. Engl. J. Med.* **354** (15): 1601–13

International Journal of Cardiology March 10, 2005; Volume 99, Issue 1, Pages 65-70

RESOURCES

Harvard Website For Low Gi Food, http://www.health.harvard.edu/newsweek/Glycemic_index_and_glycemic_load_for_100_foods.htm

The Last Four Doctors's You'll Ever Need by Paul Chek

Timeless Secrets Of Health And Rejuvenation by Andreas Moritz

Biochemical Imbalances Of Disease by Lorraine Nicolle

Why Isn't My Brain Working by Datis Kharrazian

The Book Of Ayurveda by Judith Morrison

Secrets Of People Who Never Get Sick by Gene Stone

The Blue Zones by Dan Buettner

The Okinawa Diet Plan by Bradley Wilcox

Staying Young by Micheal Roizen and Mehmet Oz

CPSIA information can be obtained
at www.ICGtesting.com
Printed in the USA
LVOW04s0333221215

467435LV00016B/1127/P